TELEHEALTH

Incorporating Interprofessional Practice for
Healthcare Professionals in the 21st Century

TELEHEALTH

Incorporating Interprofessional Practice for Healthcare Professionals in the 21st Century

KIMBERLY NOEL, MD, MPH
Clinical Assistant Professor
Family, Population and Preventive Medicine
Stony Brook Renaissance School of Medicine and
School of Health Technology and Management
Stony Brook University
Stony Brook, NY, USA

RENEE FABUS, PHD, CCC-SLP, TSHH
Associate Professor
Stony Brook University
Stony Brook, NY, USA

ELSEVIER

ISBN: 978-0-7020-8423-2

Content Strategist: Robert Edwards
Content Project Manager: Kritika Kaushik
Designer: Bridget Hoette

Printed in India

Last digit is the print number: 9 8 7 6 5 4 3 2

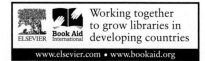

CONTENTS

v

The healthcare industry faces a pivotal moment in telehealth. As a clinical leader driving connected health innovation for the past three decades, and as Chair of the Board at the American Telemedicine Association, I have had the privilege to witness and lead the rapid adoption of telehealth. I can confidently say that the choices we make in the near future will pave the way for the decades to come. As editor-in-chief of *npj Digital Medicine*, a Nature Research journal, I promote and value the evidence base needed to guide innovation and the implementation of digital health. Textbooks such as this contribute the knowledge and academic thought that are essential to the progression of the field.

The COVID-19 pandemic exposed patients for the first time in history to the convenience of having the doctor's office brought into their home, and by all accounts they loved it. People now know what telehealth is, they have had good experiences with it, and they want to do more. However, there are strong magnetic forces pulling the provider industry back toward brick-and-mortar care unless we actively educate providers and enhance advocacy for virtual care. We have learned that telehealth should not exacerbate existing health disparities; formalized education to understand the social determinants of telehealth, as presented in this book, is important in addressing these issues. The rich content in this textbook will promote enhanced understanding of the opportunities of interprofessional practice, optimal clinical approaches to virtual care, and cutting-edge topics in the field.

It is my pleasure to know the editors and contributing authors of this textbook and to enjoy the collaboration with these national leaders in confronting our fixed place–based past in healthcare to ensure the future is paved with high-quality, convenient, and accessible healthcare. Interprofessional education and partnership is key for us to achieve these goals.

Telehealth is now a household word. Students of the field will need to lead the future, defining the right percentage of care to be delivered by telehealth, the optimal methods of telehealth practice and best ways to work among the professions to achieve the best outcomes. I hope that this book encourages the next generation of students to embrace the challenges of virtual care and to continue the path forward in telehealth education.

Joseph Kvedar, MD

Dr. Joseph Kvedar is an international physician thought leader and author who works to advance the adoption of telehealth and virtual care technologies at the national level. He is the editor-in-chief of *npj Digital Medicine*, a Nature Research journal, as well as a senior advisor of virtual care at Mass General Brigham and a senior advisor of Massachusetts General Hospital Center for Innovation in Digital Healthcare (CIDH). Dr. Kvedar serves as chair of the board of the American Telemedicine Association and co-chair of the American Medical Association's Digital Medicine Payment Advisory Group (DMPAG), which works to ensure the widespread coverage of telehealth and remote patient monitoring. Dr. Kvedar is a member of the telehealth committee of the Association of American Medical Colleges, creating tools that will enable medical schools and residency programs to integrate telehealth into the training of future practitioners. He is also a board-certified dermatologist and professor of dermatology at Harvard Medical School. Dr. Kvedar serves as a strategic advisor at Flare Capital Partners, PureTech Ventures, and ResApp Health. He is also a member of the board of several companies, including b.well Connected Health, GoodRx, and Mobile Help.

This textbook has been written to promote essential tele-health knowledge for optimal interprofessional practice. It is essential that students graduating from different health-care programs, and current clinicians, acquire the skills necessary to conduct evidence-based practice assessment and interventions using telehealth. Although there is an emerging literature that addresses subtopics of telehealth practice, this book differs from others in addressing the importance of interprofessional education and practice. It also promotes competency-based learning and introduces core principles to guide the educational trajectory, from students in training to providers active in advanced clinical practice.

Each chapter provides the reader with substantial knowledge about the telehealth process, focusing not only on introductory principles for students, but on sharing helpful material for educators and administrators beginning telehealth programs, with a focus on interprofession-alism. Given the nature of telehealth as a ubiquitous tool of clinical practice, it would be impossible for this book to comprehensively address the needs of all the different healthcare disciplines. The editors aim to introduce topics that are key in implementing telehealth practice with the core values of interprofessional collaboration, hoping to inspire further development in this much-needed area of academic scholarship.

The textbook contributors have been chosen based on their expertise and experience in telehealth, including their success in leading and managing interprofessional teams focused on collaboration.

This textbook was envisioned to provide an educational introduction to telehealth, while respecting the expansive growth of telehealth practice. The work originated from an imminent need within our own institution at Stony Brook University to rapidly adapt educational curricula to fit the needs of students graduating into a clinical prac-tice vastly transformed by the COVID-19 pandemic. The principles incorporated into this textbook have culminated in fruitful coalitions for academic development. At Stony Brook University, an interprofessional telehealth board was formed, representing diverse professions from all the health science schools, to further academic scholarship in telehealth that is pedagogically evidence-based. The edi-tors hope that current and future clinicians, instructors, and program administrators will use this textbook to guide them in mentoring students and developing telehealth cur-ricula and/or telehealth programs at their institution.

Kimberly Noel
Renee Fabus

Gil Addo, MBA
Board Member, City University of New York (CUNY) Graduate School of Public Health Foundation, CEO-Cofounder of Rubicon, MD

JeMe Cioppa-Mosca, PT, MBA
Senior Vice President, Rehabilitation, Hospital for Special Surgery, NY

Brooke Ellison, PhD, MPP
Stony Brook University, Stony Brook, NY

Renee Fabus, PhD, CCC-SLP, TSHH
Stony Brook University, Stony Brook, NY

Charles M. Fisher, PT, MPT, MBA
Assistant Vice President, Rehabilitation, Hospital for Special Surgery, NY

Suzanne Goldenkranz, BA
Telehealth Equity Director Rubicon, MD

Leslie Haas, MBA
Digital Health Strategy Manager, Stanford Health Care, Palo Alto, CA

Alexander Heromin, MD
Department of Emergency Medicine, Sidney Kimmel Medical College of Thomas Jefferson University, and National Academic Center for Telehealth, Philadelphia, PA

Lisa Howley, PhD, MEd
Department of Family, Population and Preventive Medicine, Renaissance School of Medicine at Stony Brook University, Health Sciences Center, Stony Brook, NY

Erin Hulfish, MD, FAAP
Stony Brook University Stony Brook, NY

Yuri T. Jadotte, MD, PhD, MPH
Department of Family, Population and Preventive Medicine, Renaissance School of Medicine at Stony Brook University, Health Sciences Center, Stony Brook, NY

Aditi U. Joshi, MD, MSc, FACEP
Department of Emergency Medicine, Sidney Kimmel Medical College of Thomas Jefferson University, and National Academic Center for Telehealth, Philadelphia, PA

Elizabeth A. Krupinski, PhD
Department of Radiology & Imaging Sciences, Emory University, Atlanta, GA

Edward Marx, BS, MS
Merchandising & Consumer Science Chief Digital Officer, Tech Mahindra Health & Life Sciences, Meandering Way, Colleyville, TX

Kimberly M. Noel, MD, MPH
Clinical Assistant Professor, Family, Population and Preventive Medicine Stony Brook Renaissance School of Medicine and School of Health Technology and Management, Stony Brook University, Stony Brook, NY

Karen S. Rheuban, MD
Professor of Pediatrics, Senior Associate Dean for CME and External Affairs, Director, UVA Center for Telehealth Charlottesville, VA

Yauheni Solad, MD, MHS, MBA
Medical Director, Digital Health, Yale New Haven Health, New Haven, CT

ACKNOWLEDGMENTS

Stony Brook University
Stony Brook Medicine
The Stony Brook Interprofessional Telehealth Board,
Stacy Jaffee Gropack, Dean of the School of Health Technology and Management, Stony Brook University
Kamilah Weems,
Director, Strategic Initiatives and Partnerships in Medical Education at Association of American Medical Colleges

Kimberly Noel

I would like to thank all of our contributors for devoting their time to writing a chapter in our textbook. I hope that this book will prove to be a valuable resource for healthcare students, clinicians, and administrators. I would also like to acknowledge my friends and family for their support, as well as the staff at Elsevier Publishing.

Renee Fabus

This textbook is dedicated to all of the dreamers: the future clinical leaders, who envision better healthcare systems and patient care in the new virtual world. To the generations before me, who have paved the way to my success. To Sander Michelis: my foundation, pillar, and north star. And to my family and friends for their unfailing support.

Kimberly Noel

This book is dedicated to my first cohort of students in the Speech Language Pathology program at Stony Brook University. May they always be known for their commitment to lifelong learning, high standards of professional behavior, collaborative practices, sensitivity to human diversity, and their ability and willingness to use their knowledge and skills to enrich the lives of others.

Renee Fabus

Foundations of Interprofessional Practice (IPE) in Telehealth

1

Introduction

Kimberly M. Noel, MD, MPH and Renee Fabus, PhD, CCC SLP, TSHH

> *"What is now proved was once only imagined."*
>
> *William Blake*

OBJECTIVES

1. Describe the evolution of telehealth.
2. Gain awareness of the foundational principles of interprofessional telehealth practice through review of the IPEC and AAMC competencies.
3. Define the concept of the virtual team and describe the different roles and responsibilities of telehealth providers.
4. Describe the term "interprofessional tele-board."

CHAPTER OUTLINE

KEY TERMS

Remote patient monitoring a service that uses digital technologies to collect medical and other forms of health data from individuals in one location and electronically transmit that information securely to healthcare providers

Tele-board a group of clinicians caring for a single patient simultaneously through digital technologies

Tele-consultant a clinical professional offering guidance or expertise to another clinician

Telehealth the use of telecommunications technologies to enhance healthcare, public health, and health education delivery

Tele-ICU the use of communication technologies to evaluate and treat patients in an intensive care unit

Telehealth provider a clinical professional performing therapeutic services, education, diagnosis, or counseling remotely

Tele-population health manager an individual clinician overseeing the virtual care of multiple patients simultaneously

Tele-presenter one who operates the camera and/or facilitates the telehealth visit with the patient

Tele-stroke performing stroke treatment and management using communication technologies

ABBREVIATIONS

AAMC Association of American Medical Colleges
IPEC Interprofessional Education Collaborative
RPM remote patient monitoring

ICU intensive care unit
EMR electronic medical record

INTRODUCTION

Telehealth, defined here as "the use of telecommunications technologies to enhance healthcare, public health, and health education delivery," has transformed healthcare delivery and will continue to reform how care is provided in the decades to come (Center for Connected Health Policy, 2020). The COVID-19 global pandemic accelerated telehealth adoption in an unprecedented surge of rapid innovation (Fig. 1.1) (Blandford et al., 2020; Wosik et al., 2020); however, little evidence exists regarding optimal telehealth training (Edirippulige & Armfield, 2017). This textbook will contribute to closing this knowledge gap by showcasing best practices for adoption of telehealth technology that is safe, appropriate, data-driven, equitable, and team-based, drawing on strengths of interprofessional practice and telehealth competencies.

This textbook is intended to address this need and provide an educational foundation for healthcare students and those professionally practicing on implementing telehealth. The foundation of this book is grounded in basic principles: using interprofessionalism and best telehealth practices. The book begins with an overview of core competencies in telehealth education and the virtual exam. It will introduce you to foundational principles, drawing from lessons of telehealth practice in the United States. The text will then focus on programmatic and financing principles of telehealth. We will introduce technological considerations and implementation strategies. The book will address equity and the importance of diversity and inclusion in telehealth practice, with a focus on underserved and, notably, disabled populations. Lastly, the book will describe tactical strategies to enhance telehealth education and provide an example of more in-depth clinical training on remote physical assessment.

TELEHEALTH AND INTERPROFESSIONAL COMPETENCIES

As telehealth becomes standard practice, reform of clinical training programs is required to meet the demand for these new competencies. In the United States, only half of medical education deans reported having any form of

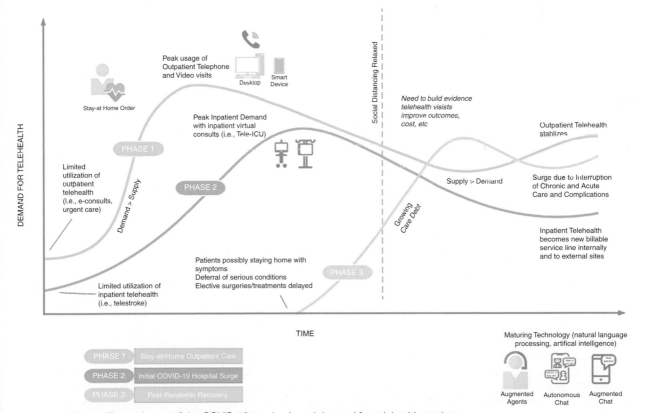

Fig. 1.1 Three phases of the COVID-19 pandemic and demand for telehealth services.

TABLE 1.1 **Interprofessional Education Collaborative Competencies (2016)**	
Competency	**Description**
Competency 1 (Values/Ethics for Interprofessional Practice)	Work with individuals of other professions to maintain a climate of mutual respect and shared values.
Competency 2 (Roles/Responsibilities)	Use the knowledge of one's own role and those of other professions to appropriately assess and address the healthcare needs of patients and to promote and advance the health of populations.
Competency 3 (Interprofessional Communication)	Communicate with patients, families, communities, and professionals in health and other fields in a responsive and responsible manner that supports a team approach to the promotion and maintenance of health and the prevention and treatment of disease.
Competency 4 (Teams and Teamwork)	Apply relationship-building values and the principles of team dynamics to perform effectively in different team roles to plan, deliver, and evaluate patient/population-centered care and population health programs and policies that are safe, timely, efficient, effective, and equitable.

Core competencies for interprofessional collaborative practice: 2016 update. Washington, DC: Interprofessional Education Collaborative.

telehealth education in the curriculum immediately prior to the COVID-19 pandemic (Khullar et al., 2021). The importance of developing a telehealth curriculum in order to deliver the "next generation of healthcare" professionals is paramount (Papanagnou et al., 2015). There are a few medical school academic programs or certificate programs that offer training in telehealth (Papanagnou et al., 2015). Many healthcare professional programs realize how imperative it is to incorporate the knowledge and skills necessary to provide services via telehealth into the professional healthcare curriculum (Cassiday et al., 2021). With rapidly increasing telehealth adoption and little foundational education available for guidance, healthcare must draw from pedagogical insight from training for in-person care and competency-based education.

Modern clinical education has incorporated models that include interprofessional practice and team-based care, which will need to be adopted for virtual care. Best practices for virtual teams can be informed by competencies on effective interprofessional practice and telehealth competencies. This textbook draws from two main bodies of work: the competencies of the Interprofessional Education Collaborative (IPEC) Expert Panel for interprofessional practice, and the Telehealth Competencies of the Association of American Medical Colleges (AAMC).

IPEC is an organization currently representing 21 national health professions associations in the United States and is a leader in interprofessional education and practice. In 2011 the founding six members of IPEC developed the IPEC competencies, which were updated in 2016 (IPEC, 2016) (Table 1.1). These have been developed as best practices and are defined by four main competencies: values and ethics, roles/responsibilities, interprofessional communication, and teams and teamwork (IPEC, 2016, 2011).

The AAMC is a not-for-profit association representing over 400 teaching hospitals and 172 US and Canadian medical schools, with a mission to improve health (AAMC, 2021). The AAMC has created telehealth competencies across a continuum of experience for medical students entering residency training in the United States, to evolve as they are entering practice, and ultimately progress as experienced faculty physicians (Table 1.2). These competencies are categorized in six domains: (1) patient safety and appropriate use of telehealth, (2) access and equity in telehealth, (3) communication via telehealth, (4) data collection and assessment of telehealth, (5) technology for telehealth, and (6) telehealth (AAMC, 2021). These competencies will be discussed in greater detail in Chapter 2. Although the AAMC competencies are the first comprehensive set of competencies for telehealth clinical practice, other professions have also described the need for standardized guidance for telehealth practice. For example, Rutledge et al. (2021) indicated that nursing requires certain telehealth competencies prior to practicing using telehealth, and Slovensky et al. (2017) suggested that healthcare professions may require a new proposed model of education to include telehealth knowledge and skills such as digital communication and telehealth communication. Expanded

TABLE 1.2 Association of American Medical Colleges Domains and Telehealth Practice	
Domain	Demonstration of advanced telehealth practice
1. Patient safety and appropriate use of telehealth. Explaining limitations and benefits of telehealth, assessing patient and caregiver access to technology and clarifying roles and responsibilities during the encounter, assessing patient risk and escalation needs.	Role-models advanced telehealth practice, understanding how to manage risk through a focus on quality improvement and evaluation of effectiveness, how to coordinate care effectively, how to escalate care when patient safety is at risk.
2. Access and equity in telehealth. Gaining awareness of one's own biases and respective implications when practicing telehealth. Understanding the effects telehealth has on health equity and gaps of care. Understanding patient-centered needs.	Role-models bias-free telehealth practice, using a patient-centered approach that focuses on overcoming barriers to care, promoting equity and access in order to reduce disparities.
3. Communication via telehealth. Developing strong virtual affinity using synchronous and asynchronous technologies, while respecting patients' privacy and environment.	Role-models effective virtual presence, using eye contact, appropriate tone, and verbal and nonverbal language, while building a relationship with the patient and (with patient consent) their caregivers or social supports.
4. Data collection and assessment via telehealth. Acquiring comprehensive history of the patient using telecommunications technologies, completing relevant virtual physical examination, obtaining appropriate patient-generated data in formulating a clinical assessment and plan.	Demonstrates how to conduct comprehensive remote assessment including remote physical diagnosis and treatment, incorporating patient-generated data when appropriate.
5. Technology for telehealth. Understanding technology needed for high-quality care delivery, explaining equipment needs at both originating and distant sites, understanding limitations of devices and comprehending risk of technology failures.	Showcases ability to use equipment, teaches how to incorporate evidence-based technologies into practice, and can enact contingency plans for equipment failures.
6. Ethical practices and legal requirements for telehealth. Understanding legal and regulatory landscape for telehealth practice, including the need for informed consent, and highest ethical and professional practice. Identifies conflicts of interest in commercial services or products.	Demonstrates compliance with laws and regulations, consistently obtains informed consent and supports patient privacy, promotes best ethical standards, and discloses conflicts of interest.

Adapted from Telehealth Competencies Across the Learning Continuum. AAMC New and Emerging Areas in Medicine Series. Washington, DC: AAMC; 2021.

competency development will be necessary to support the evolving needs of telehealth for optimal practice in the different professions (CDC, 2021).

EVOLVING HISTORY OF TELEHEALTH

Telehealth is not new to the 21st century. As novel telecommunications technologies are invented, medical applications have quickly become adopted (Nesbitt & Katz-Bell, 2018). Some historians date telehealth back to the very first telephone call in 1876, when the famous inventor Alexander Graham Bell requested his assistant, Mr. Watson, to provide first aid after an accident of spilled battery acid (Aronson, 1977). *The Lancet* as early as 1879

published justification for use of the telephone following its use in a remote diagnosis of croup and counseling of an anxious mother (Aronson, 1977). As wireless communications matured in the early 1900s, notably phone and radio, physicians in many countries were using two-way communications for clinical use cases and remote diagnosis. In fact, the earliest long-distance transmissions of electrocardiogram have been attributed to the Dutch physician Willem Einthoven in 1905, through radio technologies (Ryu, 2010). In the 1920s, medical centers such as the Hauekland Hospital in Norway, along with centers in Italy and France, performed early telehealth for passengers of nearby ships at sea and served patients on remote islands (Ryu, 2010).

Key inventions such as the television, computer, and later broadband technology were quick inspirations for remote clinical practice (Nesbitt & Katz-Bell, 2018). A key historic period for telehealth was in the 1960s, when NASA pioneered the development of telehealth for astronauts. NASA performed many demonstration projects using satellite communications for rural healthcare deliveries to test technologies for space (Institute of Medicine, 1996; Nesbitt & Katz-Bell, 2018). A historic telehealth program in the United States was a partnership between Massachusetts General Hospital and Logan Airport in 1968 for emergency response for travelers (Murphy & Bird, 1974). Subsequently, telehealth has developed rapidly over the decades, most prominently in the 1990s with the growth of internet technologies and advanced clinical applications. The early 2000s marked a period of advanced clinical innovation for telehealth, with advancements in tele-ICU, tele-stroke, and even remote surgery. In 2001 the first transatlantic robotic-assisted surgery was performed by a team of surgeons working in the United States and France over high-speed fiber-optic connections. The surgery was uncomplicated, with a successful remote gall bladder removal performed in less than an hour (Gottlieb, 2001; Marescaux et al., 2001). In addition to pioneering innovations, telehealth became an important solution for addressing the rising costs in healthcare and increased health disparities of rural underserved areas (Federal Office of Rural Health Policy, 2020). Telehealth utilization steadily increased, albeit with suboptimal implementation due to gaps in broadband access, complicated and poor regulations (including reimbursement policies), poor staff training, and technological challenges such as interoperability (Scott Kruse et al., 2018). It was not until the COVID-19 pandemic that the adoption of telehealth reached unprecedented levels.

On March 12, 2020, when the WHO announced that the COVID-19 outbreak was a pandemic, there was a rapidly accelerating number of cases and deaths in China, South Korea, Iran, Italy, and Spain. Worldwide there were 134,576 reported cases and 4981 deaths. Two weeks later, there was an increase in cases and deaths of over 300% (Fisk et al., 2020). Public health mandates required social distancing, quarantine when exposed, and isolation when infected with the respiratory virus, yet the public still required access to routine healthcare. As the pandemic ensued, there was a large risk for occupational exposure for clinicians, and nonurgent practices were closed to prioritize the needs of COVID-19 patients and to prevent iatrogenic exposures (Bokolo, 2021). Telehealth access became a key part of public health strategy (US Department of Health and Human Services, 2020). Even in underresourced settings, telehealth was seen as a strategic tool to reach those at greatest risk for viral transmission. For example, more than 68% of India's population resides in distant rural, tribal or hilly areas, representing a large unmet gap of COVID-19 screening and early diagnosis amenable to telehealth practice (Malhotra et al., 2020). In the United States, several phases of telehealth were described, as the COVID-19 pandemic created unique demands for telehealth services, including the initial phase of social distancing workflows using phone and video; a second phase increasing inpatient telehealth services, such as tele-ICU and telehealth for isolated COVID-19 patients and persons under investigation; and lastly, postpandemic preparedness, such as remote emergency care and telehealth services to address the "care debt" of neglected services that had been postponed in prioritizing the COVID-19 response (Wosik et al., 2020).

DIGITAL TRANSFORMATION: LESSONS FROM OTHER INDUSTRIES

As healthcare undergoes digital transformation, there is much to learn from other industries that have undergone virtualization, particularly businesses that are highly regulated with performance standards of enhanced security, authentication, precision, and accuracy. Remote work gained popularity as a strategy for reducing the cost of commuting, notably in the setting of rising oil prices in the 1980s (Joice, 2000). In 1996 remote work became part of many government initiatives; for example, in the United States, President Clinton's National Telecommuting Initiative was launched, co-led by the US General Services Administration and US Dept of Transportation. In the early 2000s as WiFi internet became mainstream, industries established virtual coworking spaces and began to implement telecommuting policies. In 2005 the Federal Financial Institutions Examination Council announced rules and regulations for financial institutions that established standards for risk-based assessments, customer awareness evaluations, security measures, and authenticated remote access, which drove increases in online banking (FFIEC, 2011). In 2007 Apple launched the iPhone, selling 1 million phones in a period of 74 days and experiencing astronomical sales growth estimated at over 2.2 billion phones by 2018 (Apple, 2007; Costello, 2019). With these new technologies, online businesses thrived and underwent digital transformation. By 2009 online banking had changed so vastly that the ratio of bank branches to the US population reduced dramatically, from 9340 in 1970 to 3684 in 2009 (Federal Deposit Insurance Corporation, n.d.). According to the Pew Research Center, by 2013 51% of US adults, or 61% of internet users, banked online (Fox, 2013). In the same year there were 13.4 million US citizens working at home on at least 1 day per week, an increase of 35% in less than a decade (US Census, 2013). In Europe, the adoption of online banking was very swift for many countries. According to the European Commission, 25% of adult Europeans were online banking, starting in 2007; in less than a decade, utilization doubled and by 2017 over half (51%) of adult Europeans used internet banking. Countries such as Denmark, the Netherlands, Finland, and Sweden had over 85% adoption (Eurostat, 2017). In 2018, globally, 70% of professionals worked at least 1 day a week from home, while 53% were working remotely for at least half of the week (International Workplace Group, 2018).

Online businesses and remote working have been studied in business for many decades (Morrison-Smith, 2020). Validated models have demonstrated successful methods of overcoming the physical, operational, and cultural distances created by remote work (Morrison-Smith, 2020; Lojeski, 2015). As in healthcare, businesses rarely rely on practice solely by individuals, but rely on teamwork. Essential to strong virtual teamwork is identifying roles and responsibilities, including critical relationships essential for success. For virtual teams, these relationships must diminish the factors of "virtual distance", not only addressing the organizational aspects of working in different geographies and time zones, but working to reduce barriers to communication in order to create a shared context and robust information sharing, while also enhancing team affinity. Strategies to minimize virtual distance can include judicious use of face-to face meetings early on to enhance team building, careful coordination of work to be mindful of time zones, a common context regarding real-time versus asynchronous communication, and common understanding of expectations and deliverables. Cross-functional team development is essential when working with different stakeholders and can benefit from enhanced communication practices (Lojeski & Reilly, 2020).

Many lessons from other industries are applicable when implementing telehealth, as the challenges previously described are not unique to business. Best practices in modern healthcare are delivered in team-based care models with interprofessional collaboration (Institute for Health Care Improvement, 2014; Institute of Medicine, 1999; WHO, 2008). Team-based care has become a gold standard in in-person care, and yet little is known on how to translate interprofessional care into efficient virtual clinical teams. Gordon et al. (2020) and Gustin et al. (2020) indicate the importance of communication in virtual teams as a central tenet to success.

VIRTUAL CLINICAL TEAM: ROLES AND RESPONSIBILITIES

Gleaning from lessons of industry and optimal in-person care, establishing clear roles and responsibilities may be essential to effective telehealth practice. A virtual team can consist of many different roles, and it is important to think about these evolving responsibilities as new technologies are introduced (Fig. 1.2).

The most common model of telehealth may include live or synchronous audiovisual communication between the patient and the provider directly. However, as many patients struggle with digital technologies, or may not be able to show the clinician areas of the body requiring further examination, the role of the *tele-presenter*—someone who operates the camera and/or facilitates the telehealth visit with the patient—may be needed. Furthermore, the *telehealth provider* may work directly with a patient independently during the therapeutic encounter, or may require collaboration with another clinical professional, requesting a consult from a *tele-consultant*. Modern telehealth practice may involve an individual clinician overseeing the care of multiple patients as a *tele-population health manager*. For example, in **remote patient monitoring** (RPM) programs, clinicians may be involved in evaluating data for a group of patients recently discharged from the hospital, such as their daily blood pressure, weight, oxygen saturation levels, or blood sugars. Another important model of care may involve a group of professionals working virtually on a single patient's care through a *tele-board*. The tele-board is modeled after tumor board practices in the United States, where specialists work as a group to determine diagnostic and therapeutic decisions for a common patient. Tele-board is a virtual model of simultaneous consultation optimizing synchronous and asynchronous communication technologies to facilitate care coordination among clinical professionals. Synchronous care is where the participants are available at the same moment in time to connect via communications technology such as video. Asynchronous care allows one to overcome the barriers of time by having participants interact at different moments through electronic messaging, such as use of a patient portal. Asynchronous technologies may be the use of digital messaging, stored and forwarded data such as photographs or radiologic images, or reports of a patient's physiologic parameters or lab values over time. Most commonly, asynchronous care is performed through the electronic medical record (EMR). Many modern technologies are now offering new solutions for complex data transfer for asynchronous management. The tele-board is meant to represent a chronological relationship virtually, which complements the patient's care journey or the "arc of care" representing episodic encounters with providers, to identify opportunities for digital navigation, collaboration, live virtual sessions, or e-consultations among providers (Fig. 1.3).

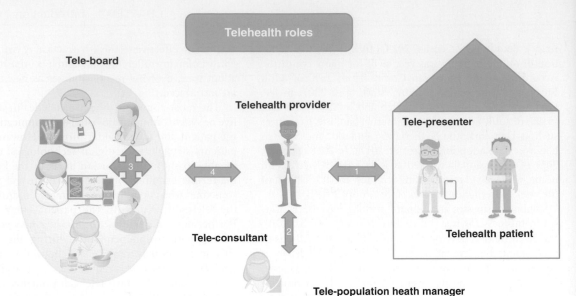

Telehealth roles

Tele-board

Telehealth provider

Tele-presenter

Telehealth patient

Tele-consultant

Tele-population heath manager

1. *Telehealth provider* connects with the patient and the *tele-presenter* who facilitates the visit by aiding the patient with remote devices
2. *Tele-consultant* is an individual who can provide remote clinical expertise to another clinician
3. *Tele-population health manager* cares for multiple virtual patients simultaneously
4. *Tele-board* is a group of clinicians working together in the virtual space using synchronous and asynchronous communications technologies

Fig. 1.2 Telehealth roles.

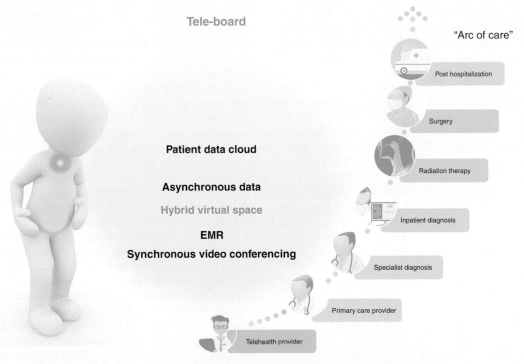

Tele-board

"Arc of care"

Post hospitalization

Surgery

Patient data cloud

Radiation therapy

Asynchronous data

Hybrid virtual space

Inpatient diagnosis

EMR

Synchronous video conferencing

Specialist diagnosis

Primary care provider

Telehealth provider

This "Arc of care" represents episodes where clinicians are interacting with the patient longitudinally over time. The hybrid virtual space represents the interactions of tele-board using synchronous and asynchronous communications technology to manage the patient simultaneously.

Fig. 1.3 Visual illustration of the arc of care and the tele-board model.

CASE STUDY: TRAINING CLINICIANS ON TELE-BOARD PRACTICE

Stony Brook Medicine has established a model called tele-board which has been integrated into clinical education, training, and practice. Tele-board is the optimization of the asynchronous and synchronous virtual space for interprofessional team-based care. The innovational education concept of tele-board is defined as the optimization of the asynchronous and synchronous virtual space for remote team care. The motivation for our tele-board initiative is to improve communication between healthcare providers and educate students about the importance of incorporating interprofessional practice using telehealth. Breakdown in communication between healthcare providers has been linked to critical patient care errors in the diagnosis and treatment of disease (Grogan et al., 2004; Kripalani et al., 2007). Ineffective communication often is the primary inciting event that leads to an adverse patient health outcome (Woolf et al., 2004). This breakdown in communication is prevalent throughout the medical care system, including the transition between inpatient and outpatient care when a patient is discharged from a hospital, leading to inadequate protection of patient safety (Woolf et al., 2004).

In order to successfully train in this virtual team model, the five health sciences schools (Dental Medicine, Health Technology and Management, Medicine, Nursing, and Social Welfare) collaborated to create the interprofessional organization in 2017 (pre-COVID-19) with the aim of training clinicians in virtual teams. The group has established an evidence-based model of telehealth care which has successfully been integrated into the education curricula for medical students, clinical training for medical residents and clinical practice of attending physicians and other healthcare professional programs at Stony Brook University. The group's mission is to create educational curricula for the healthcare programs and develop standards for the practice of telehealth across disciplines while incorporating social determinants of health.

Stony Brook's interprofessional telehealth group created interprofessional clinical cases for telehealth simulation for medical students and residents, and students in other healthcare professions including speech language pathology and occupational, dietary, and respiratory therapy. The clinical cases were based on real patient scenarios. Clinical cases simulate a patient's trajectory through multiple healthcare environments and engage clinicians from different specialties to interact in teams using both the virtual telehealth space and in-person encounters.

An illustrative example of this telehealth simulation for one of their medical student telehealth courses is a virtual case that was developed for a simulated patient suffering from dysphagia secondary to a cerebrovascular accident. The simulation followed the patient through a complex arc of care that involved an initial encounter with a primary care physician and referrals to various specialists, including a speech language pathologist, a dietitian, and a gastroenterologist, which resulted in an inpatient diagnosis of cancer, treatment of the cancer that involved the specialty expertise of a radiation oncologist and gastrointestinal surgeon, and conclusion with referral to a palliative care specialist for end-of-life-treatment. Fig. 1.3 illustrates the arc of care for a patient cared for using a tele-board model.

In addition to the medical school student curriculum, the Stony Brook Department of Medicine created cases to train internal medicine residents, including chronic pain and opioid treatment simulations for medical student training in the electronic medical record (Wong et al., 2019). Similar to the dysphagia simulation case, the chronic pain simulation followed the patient through a complex arc of care that included healthcare providers from various specialties, including primary care, pain management, psychiatry, and social work. Trainees engaged in synchronous video visits with both patients and colleagues and used the electronic medical record to respond to messages and changes in the mock EMR account.

SUMMARY

Telehealth is a rapidly developing field. Much research is required to evaluate its efficacy and the optimal outcomes for telehealth training. However, this textbook will introduce you to the expertise of telehealth leaders with advanced skills and experience in telehealth practice. The text will also introduce foundational principles and competency-based objectives to advance clinical practice. Interprofessional virtual practice is important for meeting the quadruple aim in healthcare, and students reading this book will be gaining a foundational understanding of telehealth for the years to come.

KEY POINTS

- As advances were made in technological innovations, and specifically in telecommunications and broadband, applications for clinical practice have been adopted.
- Telehealth has evolved at a rapid pace since the beginning of the COVID-19 pandemic and is a valuable tool for providing person-centered care remotely.
- The COVID-19 pandemic accelerated telehealth adoption globally at unprecedented levels in different healthcare programs.
- IPEC is the Interprofessional Educational Collaborative; it currently has 21 organizational members.
- AAMC created telehealth competencies with six domains across a continuum of care.

? CRITICAL THINKING EXERCISES

1. What can healthcare professionals learn from digital transformations in other industries?
2. What role does effective communication and teamwork play in telehealth practice?
3. What clinical professions may be involved in complex medical care like a tele-ICU or remote patient monitoring for someone diagnosed with a stroke?

RESOURCE LIST

Association of American Medical Colleges (AAMC): https://www.aamc.org/
Center for Connected Health Policy: https://www.cchpca.org/
Interprofessional Education Collaborative (IPEC): https://www.ipecollaborative.org/
World Health Organization: https://www.who.int/health-topics/digital-health#tab=tab_1

REFERENCES

AAMC. *Who we are.* https://www.aamc.org/who-we-are. [Accessed 31 October 2021].

AAMC. (2021). *Telehealth competencies across the learning continuum.* AAMC New and Emerging Areas in Medicine Series. Washington, DC: AAMC.

Apple. (2007). *Apple sells one millionth iPhone.* https://www.apple.com/newsroom/2007/09/10Apple-Sells-One-Millionth-iPhone/. [Accessed 31 October 2021].

Aronson, S. H. (1977). The Lancet on the telephone 1876–1975. *Medical History*, *21*(1), 69–87. https://doi.org/10.1017/s0025727300037182.

Blandford, A., Wesson, J., Amalberti, R., et al. (2020). Opportunities and challenges for telehealth within, and beyond, a pandemic. *Lancet Global Health*, *8*(11), e1364–e1365. https://doi.org/10.1016/S2214-109X(20)30362-4.

Bokolo, A. J. (2021). Exploring the adoption of telemedicine and virtual software for care of outpatients during and after COVID-19 pandemic. *Irish Journal of Medical Science*, *190*(1), 1–10. https://doi.org/10.1007/s11845-020-02299-z.

Cassiday, O. A., Nickasch, B. L., & Mott, J. D. (2021). Exploring telehealth in the graduate curriculum. *Nursing Forum*, *56*(1), 228–232. https://doi.org/10.1111/nuf.12524.

Center for Connected Health Policy (n.d.). *What is telehealth?* https://www.cchpca.org/about/about-telehealth. [Accessed 31 October 2021].

Centers for Disease Control and Prevention. *Using telehealth to expand access to essential health services during the COVID-19 pandemic.* https://www.cdc.gov/coronavirus/2019-ncov/hcp/telehealth.html. [Accessed 22 February 2021].

Costello, S. (2019). *How many iPhones have been sold worldwide?* https://www.lifewire.com/how-many-iphones-have-been-sold-1999500. [Accessed 31 October 2021].

Edirippulige, S., & Armfield, N. R. (2017). Education and training to support the use of clinical telehealth: A review of the literature. *Journal of Telemedicine and Telecare*, *23*(2), 273–282. https://doi.org/10.1177/1357633X16632968.

Eurostat. (2017). *Internet banking on the rise.* https://ec.europa.eu/eurostat/web/products-eurostat-news/-/DDN-20180115-1. [Accessed 31 October 2021].

Federal Deposit Insurance Corporation. (2011). *FFIEC Supplement to Authentication in an internet banking*

Environment. https://www.fdic.gov/news/financial-institu-tion-letters/2011/fil11050.html#:~:text=In%202005%2C%20the%20FFIEC%20issued,an%20increasingly%20hostile%20online%20environment. [Accessed 31 October 2021].

Federal Deposit Insurance Corporation (n.d.). *Annual historical bank data*. https://banks.data.fdic.gov/explore/historical. [Accessed 31 October 2021].

Federal Office of Rural Health Policy (FORHP). (2020). https://www.hrsa.gov/rural-health/telehealth.

Institute of Medicine Committee on Evaluating Clinical Applications of Telemedicine. (1996). Evolution and current applications of telemedicine. In M. J. Field (Ed.), *Telemedicine: A guide to assessing telecommunications in health care*. Washington, DC: National Academy Press.

Fisk, M., Livingstone, A., & Pit, S. W. (2020). Telehealth in the context of COVID-19: Changing perspectives in Australia, the United Kingdom, and the United States. *Journal of Medical Internet Research*, 22(6), e19264. https://doi.org/10.2196/19264.

Fox, S. (2013). *51% of US adults bank online*. https://www.pewresearch.org/internet/2013/08/07/51-of-u-s-adults-bank-online/. [Accessed 31 October 2021].

Gordon, H. S., Solanki, P., Bokhour, B. G., et al. (2020). "I'm not feeling like I'm part of the conversation" patients' perspectives on communicating in clinical video telehealth visits. *Journal of General Internal Medicine*, 35(6), 1751–1758. https://doi.org/10.1007/s11606-020-05673-w.

Gottlieb, S. (2001). Surgeons perform transatlantic operation using fibreoptics. *BMJ*, 323(7315), 713. https://doi.org/10.1136/bmj.323.7315.713/c.

Grogan, E. L., Stiles, R. A., France, D. J., et al. (2004). The impact of aviation-based teamwork training on the attitudes of health-care professionals. *Journal of the American College of Surgeons*, 199(6), 843–848. https://doi.org/10.1016/j.jamcollsurg.2004.08.021.

Gustin, T. S., Kott, K., & Rutledge, C. (2020). Telehealth etiquette training: A guideline for preparing interprofessional teams for successful encounters. *Nurse Educator*, 45(2), 88–92. https://doi.org/10.1097/NNE.0000000000000680.

International Workplace Group. (2018). *The workspace revolution: Reaching the tipping point*. http://contact.regus.com/GBS18_Report_Download_Request. [Accessed 31 October 2021].

IPEC. (2011). *Core competencies for interprofessional collaborative practice: Report of an expert panel*. Washington, DC: Interprofessional Education Collaborative.

IPEC. (2016). *Core competencies for interprofessional collaborative practice: 2016 update*. Washington, DC: Interprofessional Education Collaborative.

Joice, W. (2000). *The Evolution of Telework in the Federal Government. Office of Governmentwide Policy*. US General Services Administration. https://rosap.ntl.bts.gov/view/dot/14140/dot_14140_DS1.pdf. [Accessed 31 October 2021].

Khullar, D., Mullangi, S., Yu, J., et al. (2021). The state of telehealth education at U.S. medical schools. *Healthcare (Amsterdam, Netherlands)*, 9(2), 100522. https://doi.org/10.1016/j.hjdsi.2021.100522.

Kripalani, S., LeFevre, F., Phillips, C. O., et al. (2007). Deficits in communication and information transfer between hospital-based and primary care physicians: Implications for patient safety and continuity of care. *JAMA*, 297(8), 831–841. https://doi.org/10.1001/jama.297.8.831.

Lojeski, K. S. (2015). *Hidden traps of virtual teams*. HBR Webinar. [Accessed 31 October 2021]. https://hbr.org/webinar/2015/11/hidden-traps-of-virtual-teams.

Lojeski, K., & Reilly, R. (2020). *The power of virtual distance. a guide to productivity and happiness in the age of remote work*. Hoboken. NJ: John Wiley & Sons.

Malhotra, N., Sakthivel, P., Gupta, N., et al. (2020). Telemedicine: A new normal in COVID era; perspective from a developing nation. *Postgraduate Medical Journal*. https://doi.org/10.1136/postgradmedj-2020-138742.

Marescaux, J., Leroy, J., Gagner, M., et al. (2001). Transatlantic robot-assisted telesurgery. *Nature*, 413(6854), 379–380. https://doi.org/10.1038/35096636.

Morrison-Smith, S., & Ruiz, J. (2020). Challenges and barriers in virtual teams: A literature review. *SN Applied Sciences*, 2, 1–33.

Murphy, R. L. J., & Bird, K. T. (1974). Telediagnosis: A new community health resource. Observations on the feasibility of telediagnosis based on 1000 patient transactions. *American Journal of Public Health*, 64(2), 113–119. https://doi.org/10.2105/ajph.64.2.113.

Nesbitt, T. S., & Katz-Bell, J. (2018). History of telehealth. In K. Rheuban K, & E. A. Krupinski (Eds.), *Understanding telehealth*. McGraw-Hill.

Papanagnou, D., Sicks, S., & Hollander, J. E. (2015). Training the next generation of care providers: Focus on telehealth. *Healthcare Transformation*, 1(1), 52–63. https://doi.org/10.1089/heat.2015.29001-psh.

Rutledge, C. M., O'Rourke, J., Mason, A. M., et al. (2021). Telehealth competencies for nursing education and practice: The four P's of telehealth. *Nurse Educator*, 46(5), 300–305. https://doi.org/10.1097/NNE.0000000000000988.

Ryu, S. (2010). History of telemedicine: Evolution, context, and transformation. *Healthcare Informatics Research*, 16(1), 65–66. https://doi.org/10.4258/hir.2010.16.1.65.

Scott Kruse, C., Karem, P., Shifflett, K., et al. (2018). Evaluating barriers to adopting telemedicine worldwide: A systematic review. *Journal of Telemedicine and Telecare*, 24(1), 4–12. https://doi.org/10.1177/1357633X16674087.

Slovensky, D. J., Malvey, D. M., & Neigel, A. R. (2017). A model for mHealth skills training for clinicians: Meeting the future now. *MHealth*, 3, 24. https://doi.org/10.21037/mhealth.2017.05.03.

US Census. (2013). *How do we know? Working at home is on the rise*. https://www.census.gov/library/visualizations/2013/comm/home_based_workers.html. [Accessed 31 October 2021].

US Department of Health and Human Services. (2020). *Secretary Azar Announces historic expansion of telehealth access to combat COVID-19*. https://www.hhs.gov/about/news/2020/03/17/secretary-azar-announces-historic-expansion-of-tele-health-access-to-combat-covid-19.html. [Accessed 31 October 2021].

Wong, R., Carroll, W., Muttreja, A., et al. (2019). Improving opioid management and resource utilization in an internal medicine residency clinic: A before-after study over two plan-do-study-act cycles. *Pain Medicine*, *20*(10), 1919–1924. https://doi.org/10.1093/pm/pny239.

Woolf, S. H., Kuzel, A. J., Dovey, S. M., et al. (2004). A string of mistakes: The importance of cascade analysis in describing, counting, and preventing medical errors. *The Annals of Family Medicine*, *2*(4), 317–326. https://doi.org/10.1370/afm.126.

Wosik, J., Fudim, M., Cameron, B., et al. (2020). Telehealth transformation: COVID-19 and the rise of virtual care. *Journal of the American Medical Informatics Association: JAMIA*, *27*(6), 957–962. https://doi.org/10.1093/jamia/ocaa067.

BIBLIOGRAPHY

1. Wosik, J., Fudim, M., Cameron, B., et al. (2020). Telehealth transformation: COVID-19 and the rise of virtual care. *Journal of the American Medical Informatics Association: JAMIA*, *27*(6), 957–962. https://doi.org/10.1093/jamia/ocaa067.
2. Blandford, A., Wesson, J., Amalberti, R., et al. (2020). Opportunities and challenges for telehealth within, and beyond, a pandemic. *Lancet Global Health*, *8*(11), e1364–e1365. https://doi.org/10.1016/S2214-109X(20)30362-4.
3. Wherton, J., Shaw, S., Papoutsi, C., et al. (2020). Guidance on the introduction and use of video consultations during COVID-19: Important lessons from qualitative research. *BMJ Leader*, *4*(3), 120. LP – 123 https://doi.org/10.1136/leader-2020-000262.
4. Dorman, T. (2000). Telemedicine. *Anesthesiology Clinics of North America*, *18*(3), 663–676. https://doi.org/10.1016/s0889-8537(05)70185-1.
5. Center for Connected Health Policy (n.d.). What is telehealth? https://www.cchpca.org/about/about-telehealth. [Accessed 31 October 2021].
6. Malhotra, N., Sakthivel, P., Gupta, N., et al. (2020). Telemedicine: A new normal in COVID era; perspective from a developing nation. *Postgraduate Medical Journal*. https://doi.org/10.1136/postgradmedj-2020-138742.
7. Aronson, S. H. (1977). The Lancet on the telephone 1876-1975. *Medical History*, *21*(1), 69–87. https://doi.org/10.1017/s0025727300037182.
8. Ryu, S. (2010). History of telemedicine: Evolution, context, and transformation. *Healthcare Informatics Research*, *16*(1), 65–66. https://doi:10.4258/hir.2010.16.1.65.
9. Toptal. (n.d.). *The history of remote work*, 1560–present. https://www.toptal.com/insights/rise-of-remote/history-of-remote-work.
10. Bennett, A. M., Rappaport, W. H., Skinner, F. L., National Center for Health Services Research., & Mitre Corporation. (1978). *Telehealth handbook: A guide to telecommunications technology for rural health care.* Hyattsville, Md: U.S. Dept. of Health, Education, and Welfare, Public Health Service, National Center for Health Services Research.
11. Nesbitt, T. S., & Katz-Bell, J. (2018). History of telehealth. In K. Rheuban K, & E. A. Krupinski (Eds.), *Understanding telehealth*. McGraw-Hill.
12. Pilcher, J. (n.d.). *Infographic: the history of internet banking (1983–2012)*. https://thefinancialbrand.com/25380/yodlee-history-of-internet-banking/. [Accessed 31 October 2021].
13. Fox, S., & Beier, J. (2006). *Online banking 2006: Surfing to the bank*. https://www.pewinternet.org/wp-content/uploads/sites/9/media/Files/Reports/2006/PIP_Online_Banking_2006.pdf.pdf. [Accessed 31 October 2021].
14. Leonard, M., Graham, S., & Bonacum, D. (2004). The human factor: The critical importance of effective teamwork and communication in providing safe care. *Quality and Safety in Health Care*, *13*, 85–90.
15. Lingard, L. S., Espin, S., Whyte, G., et al. (2004). Communication failures in the operating room: an observational classification of recurrent types and effects. *Quality and Safety in Health Care*, *13*, 330–334.

2

Definitions and Core Competencies for Interprofessional Education in Telehealth Practice

Yuri T. Jadotte, MD, PhD, MPH, Lisa Howley, PhD, MEd, and Kimberly M. Noel, MD, MPH

> *"Interprofessional collaboration is not only possible and plausible, given what we know about how to build social capital among healthcare professionals, patients, families, and communities, how to coordinate care, and how to provide good patient care, it is also potentially self-sustaining, once it becomes a well-established component of a healthcare system and society. It may be then that interprofessional collaboration is potentially one of the best interventions we have yet conceived of to achieve the Triple Aim of improving the patient experience of care, attaining good population health outcomes, and reducing healthcare costs."*
>
> *Yuri T Jadotte*

OBJECTIVES

1. Describe the evolution of interprofessional education in medical and health professional education
2. Define the interprofessional competencies and their development in relation to major trends in health professional education
3. Explain the relationship between interprofessional education, collaborative practice, competencies, and population health in the context of telehealth practice
4. Describe how the AAMC telehealth competencies for physician training in the United States may inform telehealth competency development for interprofessional collaborative practice
5. Identify the foundational components of models of telehealth practice that incorporate interprofessional learning

CHAPTER OUTLINE

KEY TERMS

Discipline a branch of knowledge, typically one studied in higher education (e.g., sociology, philosophy, chemistry, biology)

Health outcomes the physical and physiological changes that take place in an individual's mind or body in response to prevention or treatment interventions, often referred to as clinical outcomes the healthcare arena, or as population health outcomes in the broader health arena. Examples include life expectancy and mortality, disease burden or health function (morbidity), and injury

Interdisciplinary relating to more than one branch of knowledge

Interprofessional relating to two or more members of different health professions learning together and about each other to improve a common goal in health or healthcare

Interprofessional collaborative practice the act of collaboration among health professionals by continuously learning with, from, and about each other, preferably with involvement of the patient, family, and community, to improve the quality of healthcare and optimize patient health outcomes

Interprofessional education all educational interventions or programs in which learners from at least two different health professions learn with, from, and about each other to facilitate effective collaboration and improve the quality and efficiency of care and patient health outcomes

Multidisciplinary combining or involving several academic disciplines or professional specializations in an approach to a topic or problem

Population health a mission, vision, goal or conceptual paradigm concerned with health outcomes, their distribution across different subgroups within a population, and the various factors, such as social and environmental determinants, that influence this distribution

Prevention theories, models, approaches, paradigms, or interventions implemented to avoid negative health outcomes (such as disease, disability, and death) or optimize health (such as wellness, and wellbeing) at all stages of the care continuum, often comprehensively classified into 4 sub-components (i.e. health promotion, health protection, disease prevention and disease treatment)

Preventive medicine the medical specialty whose expertise and mission are geared towards improving the health outcomes of individuals and populations via health promotion, health protection and disease prevention interventions

Profession a paid occupation, especially one that involves prolonged training and a formal qualification (e.g., medicine, nursing, social work, law), drawing from one or more disciplines or bodies of knowledge

Transdisciplinary relating to more than one branch of knowledge; often refers to members of one discipline engaging in work that is traditionally beyond their own discipline

ABBREVIATIONS

AAMC Association of American Medical Colleges
CIHC Canadian Interprofessional Health Collaborative
IPC interprofessional competency
IPCP interprofessional collaborative practice
IPE interprofessional education
IPEC Interprofessional Education Collaborative
JBI Joanna Briggs Institute

NCIPE National Center for Interprofessional Practice and Education
PM preventive medicine
QIPS Quality improvement and patient safety
RCT randomized controlled trial
TPM tele-preventive medicine

INTRODUCTION

Effective collaboration among health professionals is essential to attaining optimal patient health outcomes for in-person care and for telehealth, regardless of the setting or care delivery system. However, attainment of optimal patient health outcomes is challenged by the increasing complexity of healthcare delivery (Wolfe, 2001), ongoing health professional specialization (Irvine et al., 2002), health and healthcare inequities, the growing chronic disease burden (WHO, 2021), and the scarcity of healthcare

resources (Institute of Medicine, 2012). To face these challenges, healthcare delivery needs to be well coordinated, team-based, and patient centered to optimize patient and population health outcomes within resource constraints.

Interprofessional education (IPE) is designed to improve the competence of health professionals with regard to working in teams, communicating effectively with patients and their families, respecting and appreciating each other's unique and complementary roles in healthcare, and developing shared values that sustain collaboration to improve patient health outcomes and minimize healthcare costs (IPEC Expert Panel, 2011). In essence, not only are IPE initiatives designed to help students and health professionals achieve **interprofessional collaborative practice** (IPCP), but they have also been proven effective in improving many IPCP outcomes including student and healthcare professional perceptions, attitudes, beliefs, and knowledge about IPCP (Lapkin et al., 2013), and healthcare outcomes including reduced length of stay and better patient care management infrastructures (Reeves et al., 2008, 2013; Zwarenstein et al., 2009).

IPE has substantial implications for health education, policy, and practice in the United States (Reeves et al., 2011). On one hand, students of the health professions need to learn how to be interprofessionally competent to maximize patient-centered care, and health educators require empirical clarification on the link between IPCP and patient health outcomes in order to craft appropriate and effective educational policies (Hammick et al., 2007) and validate the utility of IPE rather than uniprofessional education in their curricula (Thistlethwaite, 2012). On the other hand, hospitals, other healthcare systems, and individual clinicians need empirical evidence about whether the implementation of IPE will improve patient health outcomes and reduce costs (Brandt, 2014; IPEC Expert Panel, 2011).

Due to significant advances in telecommunication technologies, changes in the legal landscape for medical practice, and major population health crises such as the COVID-19 pandemic, telehealth education has become a critical component of health professional education. However, the relationship between telehealth and IPE remains unclear. In particular, the role of telehealth in the implementation of health professional education and the achievement of interprofessional competency (IPC) continues to be debated. This chapter reviews and presents the evidence on the development of IPCs and their implications for health professional education in telehealth.

INTERPROFESSIONAL EDUCATION AND INTERPROFESSIONAL COLLABORATIVE PRACTICE

Interprofessionalism embodies the philosophy that when two or more individuals from two or more health professions learn with, from, and about one another and work together, there can be substantial improvements in the quality and efficiency of care, and its delivery becomes more cohesive and patient-centered (Herbert, 2005). In practice, it is sometimes referred to as interprofessional learning, interprofessional education (IPE) or interprofessional collaboration (Australian Interprofessional Practice and Education Network, 2012), but it is not to be confused with **interdisciplinary**, **multidisciplinary**, cross-disciplinary, or

multiprofessional learning, all of which stand for situations in which students and health professionals learn side by side without the added requirements to learn about and from another, and without the concrete goal of achieving collaborative, efficient, patient-centered care (Barr et al., 1999). The term *transdisciplinary professionalism* has been introduced as an extension of the term interprofessionalism (Institute of Medicine, 2014) to explain what happens in settings where health professionals adopt roles that may not be traditional to their fields (Australian Interprofessional Practice and Education Network, 2012). It too is conceptually related to but contextually different from IPE.

IPE consists of all educational interventions or programs in which students or professionals from at least two different health professions learn with, from, and about each other to facilitate effective collaboration and improve the quality and efficiency of care and patient health outcomes (Centre for the Advancement of Interprofessional Education, 2002; World Health Organization, 2010). In other words, IPE represents the sum of educational initiatives that are undertaken in order to improve IPCP (Reeves et al., 2011), which in turn is thought to improve patient care and health outcomes as well as reduce healthcare costs (IPEC Expert Panel, 2011). Examples of IPE initiatives include lectures and simulation-based activities where participants from two or more health professions are present and actively engaged in learning with and about each other for the purpose of improving healthcare and patient health outcomes (Reeves et al., 2011; Reeves, Perrier, Goldman, et al. 2013.).

IPCP is the act of collaboration by continuously learning with, from, and about each other, preferably with involvement of the patient, family, and community, in the process of improving the quality of healthcare and optimizing patient health outcomes (WHO, 2010; Australian Interprofessional Practice and Education Network, 2012). IPCP is the actualization in the real world of what is learned during IPE initiatives: it is the construct that IPE interventions are seeking to influence.

Measuring the Association Between Interprofessional Education and Interprofessional Collaborative Practice

Measuring whether IPE improves IPCP first requires an understanding of what exactly IPCP consists of, beyond its basic definition. The sheer number of tools that have been created to measure the construct of IPCP is staggering, but IPCP tools specific to telehealth practice still need to be developed. A scoping review performed by the Canadian Interprofessional Health Collaborative (CIHC) reveals that at least 128 different tools have been devised for the sole purpose of measuring IPCP outcomes (CIHC, 2012). This scoping review classified these measurement tools into six IPCP outcome categories:

attitudes; knowledge, skills, and abilities; behaviors; organizational practice; patient satisfaction; and provider satisfaction (CIHC, 2012). Some of these tools have been selected and are recommended by the National Center for Interprofessional Practice and Education (NCIPE), based on the fact that they either are readily available for use by other researchers or have been used in at least two empirical, peer-reviewed published studies, and the fact that they truly measure IPCP outcomes and not tangentially related constructs such as multidisciplinary teamwork (NCIPE, 2013). In general, these components of IPCP are considered to be the intermediate outcomes of IPE, while the distal and most prized outcomes of IPE are patient and population health outcomes (Jadotte, 2016; Johnson et al., 2020).

There are numerous tools available in the literature with which to measure the intermediate outcomes of IPE as they pertain to IPCP. There is also ample and reasonably convincing evidence in the literature to support the relationship between IPE interventions and the stated IPCP outcomes. This conclusion was reached in a systematic review of the effectiveness of IPE in university-based health professional programs, in which the authors examined the best available evidence on this particular topic (Lapkin et al., 2013). This systematic review was conducted under the auspices of the Joanna Briggs Institute (JBI), one of the leading international bodies specializing in the synthesis of the best available evidence and its translation into practice in order to improve clinical decision-making and population health outcomes globally (JBI, 2014; Pearson et al., 2005). The findings of this systematic review are very revealing, even though it focused only on the effectiveness of university-based (pre-licensure) IPE programs. Based on nine high-quality primary research studies identified, including three randomized controlled trials (RCTs), five nonrandomized experimental studies, and one longitudinal cohort study, this review concluded that overall, students' attitudes and perceptions toward IPCP can be enhanced by IPE (Lapkin et al., 2013). It does caution, however, that the evidence is inconclusive with regard to the effectiveness of IPE programs to improve students' interprofessional communication and clinical skills (Lapkin et al., 2013). Note that these are all intermediate outcomes of IPCP (Reeves et al., 2011). Fig. 2.1 depicts the relationship between IPE and the various outcomes of IPCP.

It has long been evident that IPE interventions influence learner attitudes and perceptions toward IPCP, two intermediate outcomes (i.e., attitudes and provider satisfaction). Yet for very long it remained unclear whether these endeavors teach learners the skills they need to implement in practice what they have learned from IPE. How do we know whether students and health professionals have truly attained the skills they are supposed to learn from IPE initiatives (e.g., better interprofessional communication or teamwork skills)? What,

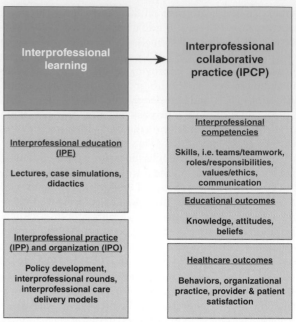

Fig. 2.1 Conceptual model of the relationship between interprofessional interventions and the outcomes of interprofessional collaborative practice, including the core competencies.

in fact, are the skills they are supposed to learn from IPE interventions? To fully understand the influence of IPE on IPCP, and ultimately on healthcare and patient health outcomes, there is a need to clearly and unambiguously define and measure how well students and health professionals have attained the skills required to practice collaboratively.

Defining the Components of Interprofessional Collaborative Practice

To address this challenge, think tanks, researchers, educators, and policymakers to date have examined the construct of IPCP thoroughly for in-person care, and have reached several overarching conclusions. First, there is a clear disconnect between the proximal and distal measures within the known IPCP outcomes (Barr, 1998; Thistlethwaite, 2012). Proximal measures examine the perceptions, knowledge, attitudes, and beliefs of students and health professionals about IPCP; in other words, the proximal measures capture the extent to which their views of IPCP have changed. Thus these proximal measures represent very subjective tools for evaluating the effectiveness of IPE activities and are generally not used as measures of attainment of IPCP (Reeves et al., 2011). Research has conclusively demonstrated that IPE endeavors are effective at changing these proximal aspects of IPCP (Lapkin et al., 2013). The distal measures, on the other hand, provide a way of identifying more objective behavioral changes in the learning environment and practice setting of students and health professionals, respectively. These include behaviors, organizational practice patterns, and other measures of IPCP. Unfortunately, these measures also do not facilitate an assessment of whether health professionals are truly ready for sustainable IPCP, as they are often self-reported (Reeves et al., 2011).

For telehealth, a similar evidence base will need to be created to track virtual collaborative practice and its outcomes. The telehealth evidence to date is large and disparate, and often relies on survey data and self-reported proximal measures such as attitudes, beliefs, and perceptions of telehealth practice (Totten et al., 2016). Not only will measures need to account for IPCP overall, but they will also need to evaluate the adoption of technology itself as part of the collaborative process. The Technology Acceptance Model explains the adoption of telehealth technologies based on proximal measures of perceived ease of use and perceived usefulness of technology, and further iterations of this model have been specified for telehealth and electronic collaboration among teams (Dasgupta et al., 2002; Tsai, 2014; Venkatesh & Davis, 1996).

Research has shown that IPE can change the distal aspect of IPCP (Reeves et al., 2008, 2013; Zwarenstein et al., 2009). However, achieving these proximal and distal IPCP outcomes is not akin to attainment of the objectives of these interventions by learners in the health professions. These objectives consist of the various facets of what it means for healthcare professionals to embody interprofessionalism, including demonstrating improved communication, well-coordinated teamwork, and shared roles and responsibilities, just to name a few (Reeves et al., 2011). The inability to measure attainment of IPCP by learners in the health professions initially made it difficult to link changes in IPCP to changes in patient health, population health, and community outcomes (Brandt, 2014). These challenges remain true in evaluating the effectiveness of IPCP in telehealth and team-based virtual care. Common constructs for reporting telehealth practice focus on patient and provider satisfaction, self-reported patient experience, technical quality, and perceived effectiveness and usefulness. The linkages between telehealth-based IPCP and patient health outcomes remain unmeasured to date (Langbecker et al., 2017).

Nevertheless, based on the large amounts of research done in the field over the past 40 years, these proximal and distal outcomes of IPE interventions for in-person care have been well defined in the literature and, as stated earlier, numerous tools have been created to measure them (CIHC, 2012; NCIPE, 2013). The issue, then, remained how to measure whether changes in the proximal and distal aspects of IPCP (which are known to be amenable to IPE interventions) are truly associated with changes within students and

healthcare professionals that will bring about sustainable IPCP (Thistlethwaite, 2012). In other words, when IPE interventions appear to change organizational practice patterns or health professionals' behaviors toward IPCP, is it truly because the health professionals have attained a certain level of collaborative practice that will be carried forward beyond the duration of the IPE intervention? In addition, can we be certain that IPE endeavors truly lead to embracing or embodiment of the tenets of interprofessionalism, such that investing time and resources to train students and clinicians via these endeavors will allow for sustainable implementation of collaborative practice?

Defining and Measuring the Interprofessional Competencies

For a very long time, this was a fundamental problem in the field of interprofessional care. Much research had attempted to define which sets of objectives or competencies should be considered interprofessional (CIHC, 2010; IPEC Expert Panel, 2011). An extensive discussion of the literature on this specific problem is beyond the scope of this chapter. However, after much debate, there is now a consensus in the United States on what these competencies should look like, via the work of the Interprofessional Education Collaborative (IPEC) Expert Panel (IPEC, 2016; IPEC Expert Panel, 2011). In essence, the concept of "competencies" has been adopted as the best method with which to objectively measure changes in the learning and practice environment for IPCP (Barr, 1998; IPEC Expert Panel, 2011). This concept is not new in health professional education and in fact had already been adopted and implemented by educational institutions and accrediting bodies in the United States (Frenk et al., 2010; Institute of Medicine, 2013), namely in response to the limitations of knowledge-, attitudes-, and beliefs-based methods of evaluating learner outcomes (Barr, 1998). The difference, however, is that prior to the promulgation of the IPEC consensus document, the concept of competencies as objective measures of attainment of essential skills for healthcare practice had been embraced on a uniprofessional basis only; that is, there were no agreed-upon competencies that could be measured for and across all the different health professions.

To address this challenge, starting in 2009, the American Association of Colleges of Nursing, American Association of Colleges of Osteopathic Medicine, American Association of Colleges of Pharmacy, American Dental Education Association, Association of American Medical Colleges, and the Association of Schools of Public Health convened the IPEC Expert Panel, charging it with the task of identifying core competencies for IPCP. In 2011, this panel promulgated a common framework for the evaluation and implementation of IPE in the United States (IPEC Expert Panel, 2011). It provided a clear definition of IPCs in the biomedical and health science professions. Using a consensus approach, four competency domains were identified: values and ethics for interprofessional practice, roles/responsibilities, interprofessional communication, and teams and teamwork. Each of these domains contained a set of more detailed general competency statements which provided additional guidance on what attainment of that particular competency actually looked like in practice (IPEC Expert Panel, 2011).

In 2016 this expert panel reconvened to update its recommendations in two important ways (Interprofessional Education Collaborative, 2016). First, the definitions of these four core IPCs were updated to reflect the growing importance of population health for health professional education (Interprofessional Education Collaborative, 2016). In addition, the IPEC panel was expanded to include additional health professional societies (e.g., social work, psychology, optometry, occupational and physical therapy), which had not previously been fully included in the initial discussions that led to the formulation of the original IPCs

(Jadotte et al., 2019a), and later expanded its representation of associations of the health professions to 21 members by 2019. Thus, by consensus of the professional school accrediting bodies of the largest and most influential healthcare professions in the United States, it is now very clear what exactly IPCP should look like within any health professional learner or practitioner. Table 2.1 lists the IPEC competencies, their definitions and associated subcompetencies, while Table 2.2 shows the chronological expansion of the progressively more inclusive membership of IPEC.

While these IPC domains and statements provide much-needed guidance for the development of new educational and practice-based programs, and for the evaluation and improvement of existing IPE initiatives, they are not in themselves tools to measure attainment of these competencies. Fortunately, there are now several validated tools that measure the attainment of IPCP based on these newly established and accepted IPCs (Jadotte et al., 2017). Table 2.3 provides a list of these tools, the original citations to the manuscripts that supported their dissemination, and their characteristics and limitations.

TABLE 2.1   IPEC Interprofessional Competencies, Their Definitions, and Associated Subcompetencies

Competencies Competency definition	Subcompetencies
Values/Ethics for Interprofessional Practice Work with individuals of other professions to maintain a climate of mutual respect and shared values.	Place interests of patients and populations at center of interprofessional health care delivery and population health programs and policies, with the goal of promoting health and health equity across the life span. Respect the dignity and privacy of patients while maintaining confidentiality in the delivery of team-based care. Embrace the cultural diversity and individual differences that characterize patients, populations, and the health team. Respect the unique cultures, values, roles/responsibilities, and expertise of other health professions and the impact these factors can have on health outcomes. Work in cooperation with those who receive care, those who provide care, and others who contribute to or support the delivery of prevention and health services and programs. Develop a trusting relationship with patients, families, and other team members. Demonstrate high standards of ethical conduct and quality of care in contributions to team-based care. Manage ethical dilemmas specific to interprofessional patient-/population-centered care situations. Act with honesty and integrity in relationships with patients, families, communities, and other team members. Maintain competence in one's own profession appropriate to scope of practice.

TABLE 2.1   IPEC Interprofessional Competencies, Their Definitions, and Associated Subcompetencies—cont'd

Competencies Competency definition	Subcompetencies
Roles/Responsibilities Use the knowledge of one's own role and those of other professions to appropriately assess and address the healthcare needs of patients and to promote and advance the health of populations.	Communicate one's roles and responsibilities clearly to patients, families, community members, and other professionals. Recognize one's limitations in skills, knowledge, and abilities. Engage diverse professionals who complement one's own professional expertise, and associated resources, to develop strategies to meet specific health and healthcare needs of patients and populations. Explain the roles and responsibilities of other providers and how the team works together to provide care, promote health, and prevent disease. Use the full scope of knowledge, skills, and abilities of professionals from health and other fields to provide care that is safe, timely, efficient, effective, and equitable. Communicate with team members to clarify each member's responsibility in executing components of a treatment plan or public health intervention. Forge interdependent relationships with other professions within and outside of the health system to improve care and advance learning. Engage in continuous professional and interprofessional development to enhance team performance and collaboration. Use unique and complementary abilities of all members of the team to optimize health and patient care. Describe how professionals in health and other fields can collaborate and integrate clinical care and public health interventions to optimize population health.
Interprofessional Communication Communicate with patients, families, communities, and professionals in health and other fields in a responsive and responsible manner that supports a team approach to the promotion and maintenance of health and the prevention and treatment of disease.	Choose effective communication tools and techniques, including information systems and communication technologies, to facilitate discussions and interactions that enhance team function. Communicate information with patients, families, community members, and health team members in a form that is understandable, avoiding discipline-specific terminology when possible. Express one's knowledge and opinions to team members involved in patient care and population health improvement with confidence, clarity, and respect, working to ensure common understanding of information, treatment, care decisions, and population health programs and policies. Listen actively and encourage ideas and opinions of other team members. Give timely, sensitive, instructive feedback to others about their performance on the team, responding respectfully as a team member to feedback from others. Use respectful language appropriate for a given difficult situation, crucial conversation, or conflict. Recognize how one's uniqueness (experience level, expertise, culture, power, and hierarchy within the health team) contributes to effective communication, conflict resolution, and positive interprofessional working relationships. Communicate the importance of teamwork in patient-centered care and population health programs and policies.

Continued

TABLE 2.1   IPEC Interprofessional Competencies, Their Definitions, and Associated Subcompetencies—cont'd

Competencies Competency definition	Subcompetencies
Teams and Teamwork Apply relationship-building values and the principles of team dynamics to perform effectively in different team roles to plan, deliver, and evaluate patient-/population-centered care and population health programs and policies that are safe, timely, efficient, effective, and equitable.	Describe the process of team development and the roles and practices of effective teams. Develop consensus on the ethical principles to guide all aspects of teamwork. Engage health and other professionals in shared patient-centered and population-focused problem-solving. Integrate the knowledge and experience of health and other professions to inform health and care decisions, while respecting patient and community values and priorities/preferences for care. Apply leadership practices that support collaborative practice and team effectiveness. Engage self and others to constructively manage disagreements about values, roles, goals, and actions that arise among health and other professionals and with patients, families, and community members. Share accountability with other professions, patients, and communities for outcomes relevant to prevention and health care. Reflect on individual and team performance for individual, as well as team, performance improvement. Use process improvement to increase effectiveness of interprofessional teamwork and team-based services, programs, and policies. Use available evidence to inform effective teamwork and team-based practices. Perform effectively on teams and in different team roles in a variety of settings.

Interprofessional Education Collaborative. (2016). Core competencies for interprofessional collaborative practice: 2016 update. Washington, DC: Interprofessional Education Collaborative. Retrieved on February 13, 2021 from https://www.ipecollaborative.org/core-competencies.

LINKING INTERPROFESSIONAL EDUCATION AND COLLABORATIVE PRACTICE TO HEALTHCARE, PATIENT HEALTH, AND POPULATION HEALTH OUTCOMES

Interprofessionalism is the new collaborative paradigm to which health professionals should adhere to help achieve optimal healthcare and patient health outcomes, yet this hypothetical causal chain is not always clear. Healthcare outcomes are the intermediate results of health promotion, health protection, disease prevention, and disease treatment interventions, the four levels of prevention (Jadotte et al., 2019b), and are related to the processes of care. A variety of theoretical frameworks have established what those outcomes consist of for interprofessional care. For example, in the Institute for Healthcare Improvement's Triple Aim framework,

the design, coordination, and patient experience of care can all be viewed as healthcare outcomes (Institute for Healthcare Improvement, 2009). The Evans and Stoddart (1990) theoretical model regards behavioral changes in either patients or healthcare professionals as healthcare outcomes. In fact, the aforementioned distal IPCP outcomes of behaviors, organizational practice, patient satisfaction, and provider satisfaction can be thought of as the key healthcare outcomes that can be affected by IPE. On the other hand, attitudes, knowledge, skills, and abilities are generally considered to be educational outcomes more than healthcare outcomes, given that they are the most proximal outcomes of IPE and are very subjective (Lapkin et al., 2013).

Healthcare outcomes, however, are very different than health outcomes. The latter consists of all the physical and physiological changes that take place in the patient's mind (if the pathology is psychological in nature) and body (if

TABLE 2.2 Chronological Expansion of the Membership of IPEC, From 2009 to 2019

Beginning in 2009 Six founding members	In 2016 Nine new institutional members	By 2019 21 total members
American Association of Colleges of Nursing (AACN)	American Association of Colleges of Podiatric Medicine (AACPM)	Accreditation Council for Education in Nutrition and Dietetics (ACEND)
American Association of Colleges of Osteopathic Medicine (AACOM)	American Council of Academic Physical Therapy (ACAPT)	American Association for Respiratory Care (AARC)
Association of American Medical Colleges (AAMC)	American Occupational Therapy Association (AOTA)	American Speech-Language Hearing Association (ASHA)
American Association of Colleges of Pharmacy (AACP)	Association of American Veterinary Medical Colleges (AAVMC)	Association of Academic Health Sciences Libraries (AAHSL)
American Dental Education Association (ADEA)	American Psychological Association (APA)	Association of Chiropractic Colleges (ACC)
Association of Schools and Programs of Public Health (ASPPH)	Association of Schools and Colleges of Optometry (ASCO)	National League for Nursing (NLN)
	Association of Schools of Allied Health Professions (ASAHP)	
	Council on Social Work Education (CSWE)	
	Physician Assistant Education Association (PAEA)	

Membership. IPEC Members, Retrieved on February 13, 2021. https://www.ipecollaborative.org/membership.

TABLE 2.3 Overview of the Characteristics of Eight Validated Tools to Measure Interprofessional Competencies Informed by the IPEC Consensus Statements

Name of tool	Original citation	Tool characteristics & limitations
Performance Assessment Tools for Interprofessional Communication and Teamwork (PACT)	Chiu, C.-J. (2014). Development and Validation of Performance Assessment Tools for Interprofessional Communication and Team- work (PACT). University of Washington. Retrieved from https://dlib.lib.washington.edu/researchworks/handle/1773/25364	• Measures the domains of teamwork and communication • Fails to capture the full construct of interprofessional collaborative practice
Interprofessional Collaborative Competency Attainment Survey (ICCAS)	Archibald, D., Trumpower, D., & MacDonald, C. J. (2014). Validation of the interprofessional collaborative competency attainment survey (ICCAS). Journal of Interprofessional Care, 28(6), 553-558. https://doi.org/10.3109/13561820.2014.917407	• Measures IPC using more than the four established IPEC competencies • May be quantifying another construct altogether
Perception of Physician-Pharmacist Interprofessional Clinical Edu- cation (SPICE)	Fike, D. S., Zorek, J. A., MacLaughlin, A. A., Samiuddin, M., Young, R. B., & MacLaughlin, E. J. (2013). Development and validation of the student perceptions of physician-pharmacist interprofessional clinical education (SPICE) instrument. American Journal of Pharmaceutical Education, 77(9). https://doi. org/10.5688/ajpe779190	• Measures teamwork and team-based practice, roles/responsibilities, and patient outcomes • Relies on self-report of learner • Does not measure all IPCs

Continued

TABLE 2.3   Overview of the Characteristics of Eight Validated Tools to Measure Interprofessional Competencies Informed by the IPEC Consensus Statements—cont'd

Name of tool	Original citation	Tool characteristics & limitations
Assessment for Collaborative Environment (ACE-15)	Tilden, V. P., Eckstrom, E., & Dieckmann, N. F. (2016). Development of the assessment for collaborative environments (ACE- 15): A tool to measure perceptions of interprofessional "teamness." Journal of Interprofessional Care, 30(3), 288-294. https:// doi.org/10.3109/ 13561820.2015.1137891	• Focuses primarily on interprofessional "teamness" • Relies on self-report of learner • Does not measure all IPCs
Interprofessional education collaborative (IPEC) competencies survey	Sevin, A. M., Hale, K. M., Brown, N. V., & McAuley, J. W. (2016). Assessing Interprofessional Education Collaborative competencies in service-learning course. American Journal of Pharmaceutical Education, 80(2), 32. https://doi. org/10.5688/ajpe80232	• Measures all four IPCs • Relies on self-report of learner
Hospital Consumer Assessment of Healthcare Professionals Survey (HCAHPS)	Jadotte, Y. T., Chase, S. M., Qureshi, R., Holly, C., & Salmond, S. (2017). The HCAHPS Survey as a Potential Tool for Measuring Organizational Interprofessional Competency at American Hospitals Nationwide: A Content Analysis Study of Concept Validity. Health and Interprofessional Practice, 3(2), eP1119. doi:https://doi. org/10.7710/2159-1253.1119	• Measures all four IPCs • Measures provider behaviors and does not rely on self-report of the learner • Psychometric assessment of this tool as a measure of IPC to date is limited to concept validity only
Resident Physician Interprofessional Collaboration Skills (RPICS)	Zabar, S., Adams, J., Kurland, S., Shaker-Brown, A., Porter, B., Horlick, M.,... Gillespie, C. (2016). Charting a key competency domain: Understanding resident physician interprofessional collaboration (IPC) skills. Journal of General Internal Medicine, 31(8), 846-853. https://doi.org/10.1007/ s11606-016-3690-6	• Does not rely on self-report of the learner • Measures all four IPCs • Unclear whether it has been fully psychometrically validated • Designed for physician-nurse interactions
Interprofessional education competency survey	Dougherty, C. V. (2016). Examining the Psychometric Properties of an Interprofessional Education Competency Survey. The Ohio State University. Retrieved from http://rave.ohiolink.edu/etdc/ view?acc_num=osu1461261243	• Measures all four IPCs, but with modifications to some subcompetencies • Psychometrically validated • Relies on self-report of the learner

the pathology is of biological origins) in response to health promotion, health protection, disease prevention, and disease treatment interventions. In the healthcare arena, these are sometimes referred to as clinical outcomes, and in the broader health arena, population health outcomes. Examples of these include life expectancy and mortality, disease burden or health function (morbidity), and injury (Jadotte et al., 2019b). These outcomes are the ultimate targets of both IPE and telehealth interventions. Based on several research studies, including systematic reviews and primary research studies (Jadotte et al., 2016, 2019a) and the results

of consensus-based methods (Institute of Medicine, 2015), the authors propose that a general conceptual model of how IPE influences clinical, population health, and systems outcomes is now evident. Fig. 2.2 depicts this theoretical model, which maps the comprehensive relationships thought to exist between interprofessional interventions and population health outcomes, as a tool to illustrate this causal chain.

As shown in this model, the complexity of this relationship emphasizes the need to account for a wide variety of factors that may prevent IPE from having an impact on clinical, population health, or systems outcomes. This

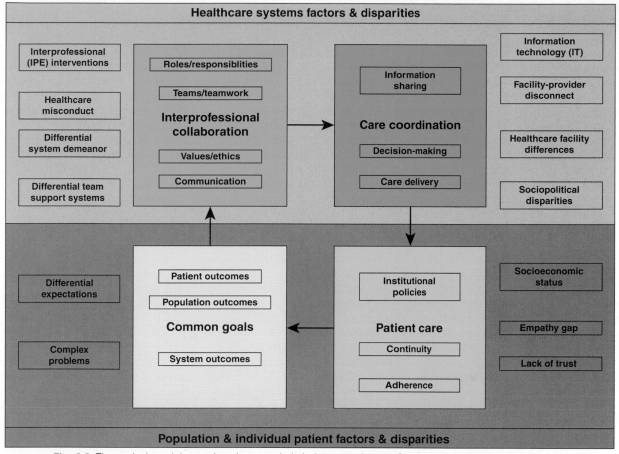

Fig. 2.2 Theoretical model mapping the causal chain between interprofessional interventions and clinical, population health, and systems outcomes.

model proposes that interprofessional interventions build the IPCs among a cohort of health professionals and improve their capacity to deliver better coordinated care, but this process can be derailed by multiple systems factors. Many of these factors are amenable to improvement by telehealth practice. For example, some of the limitations of information technology can be overcome via adequate implementation of telehealth tools. Telehealth can facilitate IPE, overcoming the time and space limitations to interprofessional learning and care delivery. Telehealth can also improve the capacity of practicing health professionals to better communicate with each other and the patient, which further improves care coordination.

Once care coordination is optimized as shown in this theoretical model, the next step in the causal chain is the provision of patient care that is continuous, holistic, and facilitates adherence, including institutional policies that are supportive of care. Here, too, telehealth has a major role to play. For example, patient care services that can be delivered via telehealth (e.g., many preventive care interventions such as behavioral/lifestyle counseling, and acute care interventions such as medication follow-ups) should be provided in this format. This can help overcome the many healthcare and social disparities that patient populations may face. Only by addressing these factors, with telehealth as one possible but major tool in the overall arsenal of the health enterprise, can clinical and population health outcomes (such as improved quality of life and increased life expectancy) and systems outcomes (such as lower healthcare cost and improved care quality) be truly achievable via IPE interventions. These aspects, as they pertain to telehealth education and practice, are further discussed in more detail in other chapters of this book.

INTERPROFESSIONAL AND TELEHEALTH COMPETENCIES: A COLLABORATIVE LEARNING EXEMPLAR

Competency-based education (CBE) is defined as an outcomes-based approach to the design, implementation, assessment, and evaluation of education programs, using an organizing framework of competencies (Frank et al., 2010). This approach has a long history in education and psychology and has expanded over the past two decades across medicine, nursing, social work, veterinary medicine, pharmacology, and other health professions. Although a detailed discussion is beyond the scope of this chapter, it is important to consider the nature of CBE across health professions when embarking on telehealth education.

The fullest realization of CBE allows learners to progress based on individual demonstration of performance instead of time or content completion. In other words, the emphasis shifts from the processes of teaching to the learning outcomes achieved. Embedded within the fullest model of CBE are frequent learner-centered formative assessments that drive mastery learning. This approach to education requires a redesign or reconceptualization of how we teach and learn.

Within and across health professions education, CBE is being implemented in various ways, utilizing different frameworks for how we envision outcomes or competencies and how we design CBE programs. Common principles of these approaches include: (1) a focus on the dynamic contemporary health and healthcare needs of society; (2) an iterative, transparent, and explicit process for translating those needs into competency statements; (3) an acceptance that achievement of competencies is variable and contextual; (4) an understanding that learning is continuous and lifelong; and (5) an understanding that learning is inclusive of formal and informal experiences (didactic, interactive, experiential) and takes place in varied settings.

The most widely adopted competency framework in medicine is the one offered by the Accreditation Council for Graduate Medical Education (ACGME) and American Board of Medical Specialties (ABMS) in 1999 (Edgar et al., 2018). This framework is now broadly adopted by other groups within and outside medicine, including the Association of American Medical Colleges (AAMC) new and emerging areas series. New and evolving demands and advances in healthcare require clinicians to acquire new competencies and continuously develop their skills. In 2017 the AAMC began development of a CBE initiative to support the inclusion of contemporary areas in medicine, such as quality improvement/patient safety (QIPS) and telehealth/ virtual care. To date, two sets of competencies have been completed and more are underway that describe expected minimum performance outcomes for medical students, residents, and practicing physicians.

The AAMC telehealth competencies (Khullar et al., 2021), like all in this series, are intended to support the ongoing professional development of physicians. They are tiered based on level of learner; integrated and built from existing competency frameworks, particularly those of the ACGME/ABMS; and applicable to all physicians regardless of specialty. The process for developing each set of competencies is similar: drafts are created based on the literature, current clinical care delivery practices, and existing educational guidelines and frameworks, and guided by leaders from across the medical education and clinical practice communities. The iterative drafting of the competencies follows a modified Delphi process (Hsu & Sandford, 2007) and is inclusive of feedback from hundreds of reactors. They are intended to add depth to specific areas in medicine and guide curricular and professional development and formative assessment. The competencies can help educators design and deliver telehealth curricula and help learners develop professionally for effective telehealth practice.

Although the AAMC telehealth competencies were developed for physicians, they share common themes with the current IPEC competencies. At the time of writing and to our knowledge, interprofessional telehealth competencies do not exist, and no other profession has defined them for their field of practice. Therefore we provide a description of these common themes in Table 2.4 and encourage further work in this educational space. This chapter defines important terms in competency-based health professions education and proposes several common themes between those defined for collaborative practice and those recently defined for medicine in telehealth. The common themes or outcomes for IPCP and telehealth based on physician practice competencies include: (1) understanding when and why to use telehealth and how to collaborate with team members in the best interests of patients; (2) mitigating biases while respecting the dignity, values, and cultural differences of patients and team members; (3) using effective communication tools, techniques, and strategies to facilitate the delivery of high-quality telehealth care; and (4) working as a team to collect and manage information and evidence to provide telehealth care that is timely, efficient, effective, and equitable. Further development of telehealth competencies for non-physician practice will need to be incorporated into future interprofessional models of care.

TABLE 2.4   Common Themes Across IPEC Competencies and AAMC Telehealth Competencies

IPEC Core Competencies for Interprofessional Collaborative Practice	AAMC Telehealth Competencies (Medicine)
Competency 1: Values/Ethics for Interprofessional Practice Work with individuals of other professions to maintain a climate of mutual respect and shared values.	Domain 4: Ethical Practices and Legal Requirements for Telehealth Clinicians will understand the federal, state, and local facility practice requirements to meet the minimal standards to deliver healthcare via telehealth. Clinicians will maintain patient privacy while minimizing risk to the clinician and patient during telehealth encounters, while putting the patient interest first and preserving or enhancing the doctor-patient relationship.
Competency 2: Roles/Responsibilities Use the knowledge of one's own role and those of other professions to appropriately assess and address the healthcare needs of patients and to promote and advance the health of populations.	Domain 1: Patient Safety and Appropriate Use of Telehealth Clinicians will understand when and why to use telehealth, as well as assess patient readiness, patient safety, practice readiness, and end user readiness.
Competency 3: Interprofessional Communication Communicate with patients, families, communities, and professionals in health and other fields in a responsive and responsible manner that supports a team approach to the promotion and maintenance of health and the prevention and treatment of disease.	Domain 3: Communication via Telehealth Specific to telehealth, clinicians will effectively communicate with patients, families, caregivers, and healthcare team members using telehealth modalities. They will also integrate both the transmission and receipt of information with the goal of effective knowledge transfer, professionalism, and understanding within a therapeutic relationship.
Competency 4: Teams and Teamwork Apply relationship-building values and the principles of team dynamics to perform effectively in different team roles to plan, deliver, and evaluate patient-/population- centered care and population health programs and policies that are safe, timely, efficient, effective, and equitable.	Domain 1: Patient Safety and Appropriate Use of Telehealth (see above) Domain 2: Data Collection and Assessment via Telehealth Clinicians will obtain and manage clinical information via telehealth to ensure appropriate high-quality care. Domain 4: Ethical Practices and Legal Requirements for Telehealth (see above)

CASE STUDY: THE TELE-PREVENTIVE MEDICINE SERVICE AT STONY BROOK UNIVERSITY

It is critical to situate IPE within the context of major trends in clinical practice, such as the rapidly growing interest in telehealth and telemedicine, and the emerging emphasis on population health as an organizing framework for driving health systems improvement. Fortunately, the refining of the IPCs to include population health as a general orientation to collaborative care has made the integration of IPE into telehealth-based care more seamless. One example of this novel integration of IPE and telehealth in health professional education is the Tele-Preventive Medicine (TPM) Service at Stony Brook University.

Launched in 2019, the TPM service is a preventive care program designed for the virtual delivery of clinical preventive services and lifestyle medicine interventions for a variety of populations, with a current focus on the patients in the Stony Brook Family Medicine Patient-Centered Medical Home (PCMH). The TPM site is a three-month rotation that provides the preventive medicine (PM) senior residents the opportunity to practice clinical preventive medicine, under indirect supervision by preventive medicine attending physicians as part of a gradated learning approach that facilitates the transition to independent practice. Clinical care in TPM takes place on Mondays, Wednesdays, and Fridays, 12:30 p.m. to 4 p.m., with virtual visits scheduled at 1 p.m., 2 p.m., and 3 p.m. For each patient, the service entails at least two

Continued

CASE STUDY: THE TELE-PREVENTIVE MEDICINE SERVICE AT STONY BROOK UNIVERSITY—CONT'D

30-minute preventive care consultations led by the PM resident with supervision by one of three board-certified PM attending physicians. Prior to or concurrent with their work in the TPM service, the PM residents actively learn the preventive services that they will deliver in the TPM service during a course run by the PM residency program, entitled "Clinical and Community Preventive Medicine." This course consists of a comprehensive overview of all evidence-based clinical and community preventive services to date, combined with monthly interprofessional case simulations where the PM residents actively engage with a practicing nutritionist, psychologist, social worker, nurse, and public health professional.

During each TPM visit, the PM resident performs a comprehensive medical history via telehealth with a focus on prevention for health and wellness, applies motivational interviewing and brief action planning (Gutnick et al., 2014) to encourage completion of desired/needed preventive services, provides prevention-focused lifestyle medicine interventions (e.g., nutrition, sleep, and physical activity counseling and prescriptions), and documents the preventive plan of care which is cosigned by one of the supervising PM attending physicians. For patients who are referred to the TPM service as part of a consult from their primary care provider, the TPM clinical note is forwarded to the primary care provider for asynchronous review. For the Stony Brook Family Medicine PCMH patient population, emphasis is placed on addressing quality metrics for which there is a gap in care (e.g., breast and colorectal cancer screening, and pneumococcal vaccination). The PM residents actively collaborate with a number of other health professionals along the course of their work leading this service, including care coordinators (most often social workers) and a cadre of nursing professionals (nursing assistants, nurses, and nurse practitioners), with interactions taking place both synchronously when the urgency of patient care demands it (e.g., prompt scheduling of a follow-up visit while the patient is agreeable to it), and asynchronously (e.g., delivery of vaccines at the PCMH clinic site days to weeks after the TPM visit).

While the TPM service currently does not bill the PCMH practice patients for the virtual visits, as would otherwise be the case under the usual fee-for-service model, it is addressing these gaps of care on behalf of the PCMH practice, which results in positive value-based reimbursements to the practice. Concurrent with the TPM rotation, residents also rotate in the Stony Brook University Hospital Employee Health and Wellness Service during the morning hours (8 a.m. to 11:30 a.m.) to further hone their skills in clinical preventive medicine. The Employee Health and Wellness service is run under an interprofessional practice model, where an attending physician, two nurse practitioners, a physician assistant, and four nurses collaborate daily to provide occupational healthcare for the Stony Brook University Hospital's 9000+ employees. The value of this approach to preventive care delivery and for optimal training in the specialty of PM has been further catapulted by the effects of the COVID-19 pandemic (Jadotte & Lane, 2021).

CONCLUSION

IPE helps health professional students and practitioners attain interprofessional collaborative practice, as measured by the four interprofessional core competencies. There is growing evidence that attainment of these competencies plays a critical role in the achievement of patient health, population health, and healthcare systems outcomes. This chapter reviewed the evolution of interprofessional education in health professional education and defined the IPCs and their development in relation to major trends in health professional education, with an emphasis on population health and telehealth practice. It offered a detailed, evidence-based theoretical model mapping the relationship between interprofessional education, collaborative practice and competencies, and population health in the context of telehealth practice. Finally, it provided an overview of one successful new model of telehealth practice that incorporates interprofessional learning, suggesting insights into the current state and joint future of IPE and telehealth practice.

SUMMARY

Interprofessional education interventions are effective at improving the ability of health professionals to work well in teams, to communicate effectively with patients and their families, to respect and appreciate each other's unique and complementary roles in healthcare, and to develop shared values that help sustain collaboration. Yet the definition and implications of these competencies for telehealth practice are still emerging. This chapter reviews and presents the evidence on the development of IPCs, tools to measure these competencies, and their implications for health professional education in telehealth. It also proposes ways in which IPCs can be incorporated into telehealth practice.

KEY POINTS

- Interprofessional education interventions are effective at improving healthcare outcomes such as patient and provider satisfaction and care coordination.
- The IPEC interprofessional education competencies, developed in 2011, have been widely adopted by nearly all health professional education programs and were updated in 2016 to reflect the increasing value of population health for the healthcare enterprise.
- Interprofessional collaboration facilitates effective care coordination and sound patient care that is holistic and continuous, leading to improvements in patient and population health outcomes.
- Telehealth practice has the capacity to help health professionals and systems overcome many of the factors that impede the successful optimization of patient and population health outcomes via interprofessional interventions, particularly the spatial and time-based limitations to care coordination and patient care delivery.

? CRITICAL THINKING EXERCISES

1. Given that it is well known that healthcare is responsible for only a small fraction (up to 20%) of positive health outcomes (e.g., diseases averted, reduction of morbidity, increased life expectancy), and that other factors such as social and environmental determinants account for a significantly larger portion of these outcomes, what role should IPE play in addressing social and environmental determinants of health?
2. IPE is fundamentally about interpersonal relationships between individuals and groups. Given what is known about these relationships from the social sciences, what theory or theories explain the mechanism by which they are developed and maintained? How does IPE actually work to improve interprofessional collaboration?

REVIEW QUESTIONS

1. Interprofessional collaboration signifies:
   a. Two or more professions working together on separate health goals for the patient.
   b. Two or more disciplines working together on separate health goals for the patient.
   c. **Two or more professions working together on the same goal for the patient.**
   d. Two or more disciplines working together on the same goal for the patient.

2. Interprofessional education requires members of two or more health professions to:
   a. **Learn together and learn about each other.**
   b. Learn together but not necessarily learn about each other.
   c. Learn about each other but not necessarily learn together.
3. A discipline and a profession relate to each other as follows:
   a. A discipline draws from one or more professions in its work.
   b. **A profession draws from one or more disciplines in its work.**
   c. Both a profession and discipline draw from each other in their work.
   d. Professions and disciplines do not draw from each other in their work.

RESOURCE LIST

National Center for Interprofessional Practice and Education (NCIPE): https://nexusipe.org
NCIPE Resource Center: https://nexusipe.org/informing/resource-center
Interprofessional Education Collaborative: https://www.ipecollaborative.org

ACKNOWLEDGMENTS

We are grateful to Kamilah Weems, Renee Fabus PhD, and Stacy Jaffee Gropack, PT, PhD for their contributions to this chapter.

REFERENCES

Australian Interprofessional Practice and Education Network. (2012). What is IPE/IPL/IPP?

Barr, H. (1998). Competent to collaborate: Towards a competency-based model for interprofessional education. *Journal of Interprofessional Care, 12*(2), 181–187. https://doi.org/10.3109/13561829809014104.

Barr, H., Hammick, M., Koppel, I., et al. (1999). Evaluating interprofessional education: Two systematic reviews for health and social care. *British Educational Research Journal, 25*(4), 533–544. https://doi.org/10.1080/0141192990250408.

Brandt, B. F. (2014, January). Update on the US national center for interprofessional practice and education. *Journal of Interprofessional Care, 28*, 5–7. https://doi.org/10.3109/13561820.2013.852365.

Center for the Advancement of Interprofessional PE. (2002). *Interprofessional Education- Today, Yesterday and Tomorrow (Barr, H.) Higher Education Academy, Learning & Teaching Support Network for health Sciences & Practice.* https://www.caipe.org/resources/publications/caipe-publications/caipe-2002-interprofessional-education-today-yesterday-to-morrow-barr-h.

Canadian Interprofessional Health Collaborative. (2010). *A national interprofessional competency framework.* https://phabc.org/wp-content/uploads/2015/07/CIHC-National-Interprofessional-Competency-Framework.pdf.

Canadian Interprofessional Health Collaborative. (2012). *Inventory of quantitative tools measuring interprofessional education and collaborative practice outcomes.*

Dasgupta, S., Granger, M., & McGarry, N. (2002). User acceptance of E-collaboration technology: An extension of the technology acceptance model. *Group Decision and Negotiation, 11*(2), 87–100. https://doi.org/10.1023/A:1015221710638.

Davis, F. D. (1989). Technology acceptance model: Tam. In M. N. Al-Suqri, & A. S. Al-Aufi (Eds.), *Information seeking behavior and technology adoption.* Hershey, PA. (pp. 205–219).

Edgar, L., Roberts, S., & Holmboe, E. (2018). Milestones 2.0: A step forward. *Journal of Graduate Medical Education, 10*, 367–369. https://doi.org/10.4300/JGME-D-18-00372.1.

Evans, R. G., & Stoddart, G. L. (1990). Producing health, consuming health care. *Social Science & Medicine, 31*(12), 1347–1363. https://doi.org/10.1016/0277-9536(90)90074-3.

Frank, J. R., Snell, L. S., Cate, O. T., et al. (2010). Competency-based medical education: Theory to practice. *Medical Teacher, 32*(8), 638–645. https://doi.org/10.3109/0142159X.2010.501190.

Frenk, J., Chen, L., Bhutta, Z. A., et al. (2010). Health professionals for a new century: Transforming education to strengthen health systems in an interdependent world. *Lancet (London, England), 376*(9756), 1923–1958. https://doi.org/10.1016/S0140-6736(10)61854-5.

Gutnick, D., Reims, K., Davis, C., et al. (2014). Brief action planning to facilitate behavior change and support patient self-management. *Journal of Clinical Outcomes Management, 21*, 17–29.

Hammick, M., Freeth, D., Koppel, I., et al. (2007). A best evidence systematic review of interprofessional education: BEME guide no. 9. *Medical Teacher, 29*(8), 735–751. https://doi.org/10.1080/01421590701682576.

Herbert, C. P. (2005). Changing the culture: Interprofessional education for collaborative patient-centred practice in Canada. *Journal of Interprofessional Care*, 1–4. https://doi.org/10.1080/13561820500081539.

Hsu, C.-C., & Sandford, B. A. (2007). The Delphi technique: Making sense of consensus. *Practical Assessment, Research and Evaluation, 12*(1), 10.

Institute for Healthcare Improvement. (2009). *The triple aim: Optimizing health, care, and cost.* http://www.ihi.org/Engage/Initiatives/TripleAim/Documents/BeasleyTripleAim_ACHEJan09.pdf.

Institute of Medicine. (2012). *Best care at lower cost: The Path to continuously learning health care in America.* National Academy of Sciences, National Academy. http://www.nap.edu/openbook.php?record_id=9780309213444internal-pdf://9783278659877/9780309213444.pdf.

Institute of Medicine. (2013). *Interprofessional education for collaboration: Learning how to improve health from interprofessional models across the continuum of education to practice: Workshop summary.* http://www.nap.edu/download.php?record_id=13486. [Accessed 11 April 2014].

Institute of Medicine. (2014). *Establishing transdisciplinary professionalism for improving health outcomes: Workshop summary.*

Institute of Medicine. (2015). *Measuring the impact of interprofessional education on collaborative practice and patient outcomes: Workshop summary.*

IPEC. (2011). *Core competencies for interprofessional collaborative practice: Report of an expert panel.* Washington, DC: Interprofessional Education Collaborative.

IPEC. (2016). *Core competencies for interprofessional collaborative practice: 2016 update.* Washington, DC: Interprofessional Education Collaborative.

Irvine, R., Kerridge, I., McPhee, J., et al. (2002). Interprofessionalism and ethics: Consensus or clash of cultures? *Journal of Interprofessional Care, 16*(3), 199–210. https://doi.org/10.1080/13561820220146649.

Jadotte, Y. T. (2016). *Understanding the association between interprofessional collaborative practice and patient health outcomes in urban settings: A mixed methods study.* (PhD Dissertation). Rutgers University and New Jersey Institute of Technology. Rutgers University Press.

Jadotte, Y., Chase, S., Qureshi, R., et al. (2017). The HCAHPS survey as a potential tool for measuring organizational interprofessional competency at American hospitals nationwide: A content analysis study of concept validity. *Health and Interprofessional Practice, 3*, eP1119. https://doi.org/10.7710/2159-1253.1119.

Jadotte, Y., Gayen, S., Chase, S., et al. (2019a). Interprofessional collaboration and patient health outcomes in urban disadvantaged settings: A grounded theory study. *Health Interprofessional Practice and Education, 3*, 1185. https://doi.org/10.7710/1185.

Jadotte, Y. T., Holly, C., Chase, S. M., et al. (2016). Interprofessional collaborative practice and patient health outcomes in urban settings: A qualitative systematic review. In C. Holly, S. W. Salmond, & M. Saimbert (Eds.), *Comprehensive systematic review for advanced practice nursing* (2nd ed.) (pp. 425–447). New York: Spring Publishing Company.

Jadotte, Y. T., & Lane, D. S. (2021). Core functions, knowledge bases and essential services: A proposed prescription for the evolution of the preventive medicine specialty. *Preventive Medicine, 143,* 106286. https://doi.org/10.1016/j.ypmed.2020.106286.

Jadotte, Y. T., Leisy, H. B., Noel, K., et al. (2019b). The emerging identity of the preventive medicine specialty: A model for the population health transition. *American Journal of Preventive Medicine, 56*(4), 614–621. https://doi.org/10.1016/j.amepre.2018.10.031.

Joanna Briggs Institute. (2020). *JBI reviewers manual.* Retrieved August 11, 2014 https://synthesismanual.jbi.global.

Johnson, S. B., Fair, M. A., Howley, L. D., et al. (2020). Teaching public and population health in medical education: An evaluation framework. *Academic medicine. Academic Medicine, 95*(12), 1853–1863. https://doi.org/10.1097/ACM.0000000000003737.

Khullar, D., Mullangi, S., Yu, J., et al. (2021). The state of telehealth education at U.S. medical schools. *Healthcare (Amsterdam, Netherlands), 9*(2), 100522. https://doi.org/10.1016/j.hjdsi.2021.100522.

Langbecker, D., Caffery, L. J., Gillespie, N., et al. (2017). Using survey methods in telehealth research: A practical guide. *Journal of Telemedicine and Telecare, 23*(9), 770–779. https://doi.org/10.1177/1357633X17721814.

Lapkin, S., Levett-Jones, T., & Gilligan, C. (2013). A systematic review of the effectiveness of interprofessional education in health professional programs. *Nurse Education Today, 33*(2), 90–102. https://doi.org/10.1016/j.nedt.2011.11.006.

National Center for Interprofessional Practice and Education. (2013). Measurement Instruments. *Interprofessional education and learning: Measurement Instruments.* Retrieved from https://nexusipe.org/measurement-instruments.

Pearson, A., Wiechula, R., Court, A., et al. (2005). The JBI model of evidence-based healthcare. *International Journal of Evidence-Based Healthcare, 3*(8), 207–215. https://doi.org/10.1111/j.1479-6988.2005.00026.x.

Reeves, S., Goldman, J., Gilbert, J., et al. (2011). A scoping review to improve conceptual clarity of interprofessional interventions. *Journal of Interprofessional Care, 25*(3), 167–174. https://doi.org/10.3109/13561820.2010.529960.

Reeves, S., Perrier, L., Goldman, J., et al. (2013). Interprofessional education: Effects on professional practice and healthcare outcomes (update). *Cochrane Database of Systematic Reviews, 2013*(3), CD002213. https://doi.org/10.1002/14651858.CD002213.pub3.

Reeves, S., Zwarenstein, M., Goldman, J., et al. (2008). Interprofessional education: Effects on professional practice and health care outcomes. *Cochrane Database of Systematic Reviews,* (1), CD002213. https://doi.org/10.1002/14651858.CD002213.pub2.

Thistlethwaite, J. (2012). Interprofessional education: A review of context, learning and the research agenda. *Medical Education, 46*(1), 58–70. https://doi.org/10.1111/j.1365-2923.2011.04143.x.

Totten, A. M., Womack, D. M., Eden, K. B., et al. (2016). *Telehealth: Mapping the evidence for patient outcomes from systematic reviews.* Agency for Healthcare Research and Quality (US).

Tsai, C.-H. (2014). Integrating social capital theory, social cognitive theory, and the technology acceptance model to explore a behavioral model of telehealth systems. *International Journal of Environmental Research and Public Health, 11*(5), 4905–4925. https://doi.org/10.3390/ijerph110504905.

Venkatesh, V., & Davis, F. D. (1996). A model of the antecedents of perceived ease of use: Development and test. *Decision Sciences, 27*(3), 451–481.

WHO. (2010). *Framework for Action on Interprofessional Education & Collaborative Practice.* https://www.who.int/publications/i/item/framework-for-action-on-interprofessional-education-collaborative-practice.

WHO. (2021). *Noncommunicable diseases.* From https://www.who.int/health-topics/noncommunicable-diseases#tab=tab_1.

Wolfe, A. (2001). Institute of medicine report: Crossing the quality chasm: A new health system for the 21st century. *Policy Politics & Nursing Practice, 2*(3), 233–235.

Zwarenstein, M., Goldman, J., & Reeves, S. (2009). Interprofessional collaboration: Effects of practice-based interventions on professional practice and healthcare outcomes. *Cochrane Database of Systematic Reviews,* (3), CD000072. https://doi.org/10.1002/14651858.CD000072.pub2.

Core Competency in Virtual Physical Exam

Alexander Heromin, MD and Aditi U. Joshi, MD, MSc, FACEP

OBJECTIVES

1. Understand the background of telehealth physical exam and current research.
2. Understand the types of telehealth being practiced and the physical exam components that are necessary.
3. Evaluate the types of training currently available for learners and what is necessary for future clinical education.
4. Identify the key components of the physical exam and which portions can be done by telehealth.

CHAPTER OUTLINE

KEY TERMS

Asynchronous telehealth medical encounters or medical information gathering done through technology not in real time

Clinical tele-presenter medical professional conducting the virtual telehealth encounter

Medical education the education related to training to be a medical provider in various roles

Remote consults medical consults conducted by providers on patients virtually or not in the same physical space as the patient

Synchronous medical encounters with the provider and patient both being present in real time

Telehealth a broader and more inclusive term encompassing not only providing services to the ill or wounded patient but also screening, prevention, maintenance, and follow-up services.

Telemedicine conducting a medical encounter when there is a sick or injured patient through various means of technology

Virtual care medical care of various scopes provided remotely or not in the same physical space as the patient

Virtual encounter a medical encounter conducted by a medical provider through various means of technology

Virtual physical exam a physical exam conducted by a medical provider virtually through various means of technology

Webside manner the way in which a medical provider interacts with a patient through technology

INTRODUCTION

Telehealth, the use of technology to have a virtual medical encounter, has expanded tremendously over the last few years, no time more so than during the COVID-19 pandemic (CDC, 2020). The substantial increase in virtual visits and use cases has created an urgent need to understand the components of the physical exam that are relevant to telehealth. These needs extend not only to the practicing clinician wanting to expand their practice but also to learners in the different stages of their medical careers and administrators that are creating or expanding their programs.

This chapter aims to outline the core competencies of current clinical practice and which sections of the physical exam can be currently converted to telehealth. It will also give an overview of the ways it is practiced in urgent care, primary care, and emergency care. We will mention adjunct devices that will be needed to augment physical exam components and the ways in which existing education needs to be updated for the future evolving healthcare system. We aim to give tangible, evidence-based ways to do the physical exam to enhance and have effective virtual care encounters.

For this section, we are using video **virtual care** as the standard due to the need for visualization, and will be going over virtual physical exams done at the patient's home. In general, these recommendations can be done without adjunct devices and we will specify when such devices need to be utilized. For the purposes of this chapter, the term "clinician" will be used to describe all types of medical clinical staff, including physicians, advanced practice providers (APPs), nurses, medical technicians, physical and occupational therapists, and any other type of staff who are practicing clinical encounters. We recognize that these other clinicians learn and practice different exams relevant to their fields. This chapter will then use the standard for medical education exam for use in telehealth.

BACKGROUND

The components of physical exam are taught in medical education as part of the preclinical years in order for students to be prepared for clinical rotations. The core standards, competencies, and curriculum for future doctors are set by the Liaison Committee for Medical Education (LCME) (LCME, 2011). These standards are taught in undergraduate medical education by various methods, and stress practical components. The set competencies allow for standardization of education across medical education.

Telehealth, reported to deliver patient care at low cost and high efficiency with high patient satisfaction across several specialties while overcoming great geographic distances, has been expanding over the last decade (National Quality Forum, 2017; Shigekawa et al., 2018). As these potential benefits of telehealth become more apparent, organizations and academic centers have begun to develop their own telehealth programs at increasing rates. In order to prepare their staff, many had to create their own training as well as research. The majority of outcome-based telemedicine studies are conducted within an academic institution where telemedicine providers are considered "experts in telehealth" or were trained by experts using modalities including lectures, videos, online modules, demonstrations, or hands-on practice (Carvalho et al., 2019; Flodgren et al., 2015; Shigekawa et al., 2018). The physicians, institutions, and companies had to create the basics of webside manner, ensure secure platforms, handle technology troubleshooting, and develop basics of how to do virtual visits, including telehealth physical exam.

Initially, most programs did not have formal virtual physical exam training for their providers. Additionally, several papers have noted inconsistencies within telehealth research, with a resulting lack of standardization and research in telemedicine education and training (Flodgren et al., 2015; Shigekawa et al., 2018). The few training programs that existed were either created for internal training or did not include physical exam training. The first course noted for this express purpose was created in 2017 by Thomas Jefferson University (National Quality Forum, 2017) and was available for CME in 2018. During the COVID-19 pandemic, an influx of programs and companies also started expanding their telehealth visit coverage in order to offer virtual services to decrease exposure and increase healthcare access (Cao et al., 2020; Chen et al., 2020; Jee et al., 2020; Spina et al., 2020; Wennmann et al., 2020; Whiteside et al., 2020). This resulted in acute interest in understanding practical components and assurance of a quality visit. Other virtual exam teaching programs and papers also emerged in 2020 to fill some of that need (Al Hussona et al., 2020; Ansary et al., 2021; Benziger et al., 2021; Stanford University, 2020; Wahezi et al., 2020).

In order to critically examine the effectiveness of telehealth virtual exam, it will be necessary to investigate whether the principles of delivering care through technology are using evidence-based teaching models for effective visits. This will be essential in the future in order to standardize care and improve the effectiveness and outcomes of telehealth virtual exam.

USE OF PHYSICAL EXAM

Physical exam components over telehealth are essentially used in a similar way over the various types of virtual visits with slight differences depending on who is initiating the call.

Provider-to-Provider Telehealth

Provider-to-provider consults generally take place within two clinical environments using two medically trained providers. A common example is tele-stroke where a "spoke" remote hospital can initiate a consult call with a neurologist or neurosurgeon at a "hub" or centralized hospital (Demaerschalk et al., 2017). The consultation is then done remotely. In these cases, the exam is being aided by a clinical provider, whether a physician, APP, or a clinical tele-presenter who is another medical professional trained in the needed exam (Sikka et al., 2021).

The use of telehealth in these situations is easier to understand as the exam is done by a medically trained professional. The receiving or consulting provider can ask questions, get information from another trained provider, and evaluate the exam techniques and patient visually. In these cases, the training for a physical exam is specific to the type of exam needed—meaning the tele-consult team are required to know and be trained in their specific roles, including how to do the physical exam on site while under guidance of the remote consultant. In the tele-stroke example, all providers and clinical tele-presenters are trained in the neurological and stroke exam and its use virtually. This has led to successes involving reduced transfers, time to tissue plasminogen activator, and outcomes (Brecthel et al., 2018; Chaffin et al., 2019; Ochiai et al., 2020).

Of note, these provider-to-provider consultations can also be done within the same hospital (Hemingway et al., 2020; Hron et al., 2020; Lau et al., 2020; SAEM, n.d.). During the COVID-19 pandemic, many institutions created a protocol for consultants to be able to do remote consults using an iPad or other virtual modalities within the hospital to decrease contagion and save PPE (Hamm et al., 2020; Redford, 2020; Wittbold et al., 2020).

One of the potential gaps is that, while observing the exam, the trained specialist is not doing their own exam and is dependent on others on site. However, it should be noted that traditionally, consultations require that the history, results, and exam components are reported by the initiating provider to the consultant over the telephone to determine the next step of care. This has always required trusting and using the information given by the other provider. Doing tele-consults may actually give more information, since the workflows and process can be planned in advance. This aspect of the virtual encounters also allows the consultant to correct or modify the physical exam techniques being done by the proxy in real time, allowing for a more thorough and expanded exam as they see fit (Figs. 3.1-3.5).

To offset the increasing number of emergency department (ED) visits, tele-triage programs have emerged for triaging patients remotely. Patients who present to the ED are placed in a room, triaged, and then have a first provider encounter virtually. This allows orders to be placed and the patient then goes through the rest of their ED visit. In some cases, an RN or tech are also present (Joshi et al., 2020). This became more widespread during the pandemic due to the

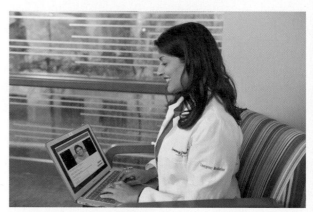
Fig. 3.1 Tele-triage programs. (Thomas Jefferson University Photography Services)

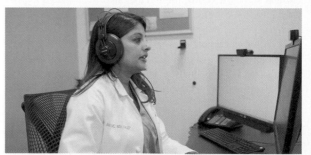
Fig. 3.2 Tele-triage programs. (Thomas Jefferson University Photography Services)

need of decreasing exposure (Chauhan et al., 2020; Grange et al., 2020; Turer et al., 2020). Tele-triage programs, while different from provider-to-provider consults, also take place with the patient in a standard clinical environment, namely the ED, and so the physical exam components are done in a similar manner (Izzo et al., 2018). Of note, there is some likely decreased use of physical exam virtually if the tele-triage telehealth provider knows the patient will see someone in person later in the encounter (Joshi et al., 2020b).

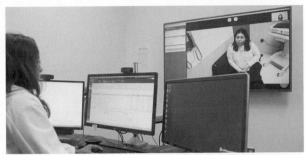

Fig. 3.3 Dr. Aditi U. Joshi assessing and conversing with a patient remotely. (Thomas Jefferson University Photography Services)

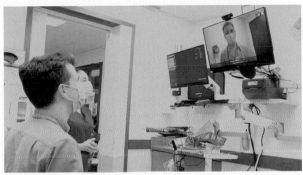

Fig. 3.4 A patient's perspective during the tele-triage intake process. (Thomas Jefferson University Telehealth Department)

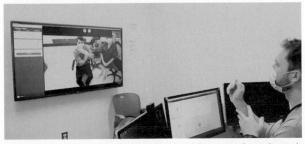

Fig. 3.5 Dr. Alex Heromin remotely guiding a patient through palpation of the wrist during the intake process. (Thomas Jefferson University Telehealth Department)

On-Demand/Direct-to-Consumer Applications

The patient-initiated acute care calls or direct-to-consumer (DTC) calls are generally done from the patient's home or other personal space (work, family member's home, etc.) (Uscher-Pines et al., 2016). By its nature, the exam is remote and will require input by the patient or the help of family members or others in the home. While many educators note that history is the most essential part of a medical encounter (Centor, 2007), physical exams are still necessary for clinical judgment. The lack of a trained medical professional on the patient side requires the patient, family, or care partner to be involved more heavily. Some research states that this may lead to overprescribing of antibiotics, lack of concordance in exam, and resulting poor-quality care (Akhtar et al., 2018; Handschu et al., 2003; Shi et al., 2018). However, others also point to improved antibiotic stewardship and reliance on quality assurance processes (Davis et al., 2019; Halpren-Ruder et al., 2019; Johnson et al., 2019; Novara et al., 2020; Rastogi et al., 2020). The need for improving home-based healthcare by increased training and standardization thus becomes crucial.

In general, home-based virtual care does require more patient involvement. The provider can ask the patient to move around, open their mouth, angle the camera, ensure the best lighting, and do whatever part of the exam as directed by the provider. Patients can also use home devices that can add to the vital signs, take their own pulse under guidance, and add any information they may have. If there is someone else to help with the exam, under provider **guidance**, they can do the exam itself. It is recognized that physicians and other types of providers learn how to do physical exam in a controlled, standardized environment (AAMC, 2021). With experience, physical exam helps the provider use that information to determine the next actionable step. In a virtual visit, the clinician relies on someone who is not medically trained; however, the clinician can likely still determine the next step. Even an exam run by a patient or family member gives the provider more information and allows the patient to understand what is important, what is a red flag, and when they may need a higher level of care (Benziger et al., 2021).

A common question is whether parts of the exam done by patients or others can be compared at all to the exam being done with one's own hands. That decision should be considered in light of the other information during the visit; if the provider still has high suspicion of worsening conditions and is not sure the exam gives them the comfort to monitor at home, there is always the opportunity to refer in for a higher level of care.

We will briefly mention the special situations when there *are* clinically trained professionals available. As telehealth expands, and prehospital care and home nursing has the capability to involve a provider via telehealth capabilities, the comfort of at-home exams may expand. These providers do have medical training, have tools to get vitals, can come to the home with devices and tools, and can gather other information in a home environment to perform the exam as needed. There may be sections that still need provider guidance; however, this type of care may be able to increase the extent of virtual physical exam. Further research and investigation of these types of visits will be an interesting addition to the current literature.

Scheduled Visits

Scheduled visits are differentiated from DTC visits simply by the fact that the patient does not initiate these visits when there is an acute care issue; instead, these are appointments that have been scheduled in advance (Powell et al., 2018). Some of the common scheduled visit types include discussion of testing results, postoperative visits, chronic care, preventive care, or other types of primary and follow-up care. For this reason, the components of the exam and history would be similar to DTC applications done in the patient's personal environment. One salient difference is that, because these types of patients are known to their physician and the visit is planned in advance, there is a role and place to extend the type of devices and applications that can be accessed at home. Along with their physician, patients can plan for telehealth visits and have the information handy, whether it is data from their home devices, vital signs or information specific to their chronic disease such as weights, blood sugars, mental status, or wound appearance (O'Connor et al., 2016; Reid et al., 2018; Xu et al., 2018).

Due to being able to plan home care for chronic needs, a dedicated team can be trained in telehealth as well as how to aid in home healthcare. This team can include, but is not limited to, the provider, patient, family, care partners, and home health aides. This advance planning can especially aid those who have more needs, are at high risk of rehospitalization, or are limited in travel for various reasons. Using telehealth can provide convenient care for patients, allow for increased follow-up and more information when following up at home with use of adjunct information, and allow for improved solutions and care planning.

Scheduled visits in cases of new patients, those without long-standing chronic conditions, or those who require a simple follow-up may not have this careful advance planning (because they are new patients, or because such planning simply is not necessary). In these cases, the type of exam done would be similar to other visits with less other information at hand. However, even these visits have the advantage of being known about in advance, so the provider and team can reach out a few days prior to ask patients to be prepared.

All of these situations beg the question of how to train patients and their care partners at the home. When we ask patients to be involved in their care, tip sheets may be required for them to understand how to best make use of their telehealth visits and involve others. This extension of training and educating as we consider the expanding home healthcare team is intriguing and can increase healthcare access significantly (Reed et al., 2020).

EDUCATION AND TRAINING FOR VIRTUAL PHYSICAL EXAM

As healthcare providers consider providing telehealth services, there is a need to ensure that they have the skills needed to effectively and safely utilize this modality of providing care. In 2014 more than half the respondents to a national survey of family practitioners reported training as a key barrier to telehealth adoption (Moore et al., 2017). Prior to the COVID-19 pandemic of 2020, telehealth programs were developed slowly with regard to the various aspects required for success, including training (Bonney et al., 2015; Edirippulige & Armfield, 2017; Hart et al., 2018; Jonas et al., 2019; Pathipati et al., 2016). During the rapid adoption of telehealth for COVID-19, there was a need for quick training for practitioners to learn effective practice over telehealth. While most studies and programs are for all types of telehealth training, some providers have hesitations or concerns about the physical exam aspect specifically, and this type of training and education is especially relevant. Despite this need, there are few validated training programs for telehealth and there is no consensus on training skills and competencies.

The American Academy of Medical Colleges (AAMC) created a list of competencies for telehealth education to alleviate some of the lack in standardization. The guidelines are in six domains and cover various levels of training, including physicians entering residency, recent graduates entering practice, and experienced faculty physicians (AAMC, 2021). Domain IV, Data Collection and Assessment via Telehealth, is relevant to physical exam and is outlined in Box 3.1.

This section will talk about the types of training currently available, what types of learners are necessary to train and at what level, and the process of validating our education programs.

Level of Learner

It is incorrect to assume that because a provider has experience with technology, this translates to an effective telehealth visit (Pathipati et al., 2016). As one delivers care remotely, the need for special attention to digital communication skills and performing a physical exam without

---

BOX 3.1 AAMC Telehealth Competencies Domain IV: Data Collection and Assessment Via Telehealth

2a. Conducts appropriate physical examination or collects relevant data on clinical status during a (real or simulated) telehealth encounter including guiding the patient or tele-presenter	2b. Conducts appropriate physical examination and collects relevant data on clinical status during a telehealth encounter including guiding the patient and/or tele-presenter	2c. Role models and teaches the skills required to perform a physical examination during a telehealth encounter, including guiding the patient and/or tele-presenter

AAMC. (2021). *Telehealth competencies across the learning continuum*. AAMC New and Emerging Areas in Medicine Series. Washington, DC: AAMC.

---

laying hands on the patient place the provider in an unfamiliar situation compared with the skills acquired in formal **medical education** (DeJong et al., 2015). Therefore the ideal telemedicine education is not specific to one specialty, but rather comprises a set of core fundamental skills that can be delivered uniformly across training programs at different levels and adjusted to a particular medical discipline (Slovensky et al., 2017).

For physicians, medical education typically includes medical student or undergraduate medical education (UME), resident or graduate medical education (GME), postgraduate training or fellowship, and training and continuing medical education of attending and faculty physicians. Clinicians of other professions must also be proficient in telehealth services relevant to their degree and role in the clinical encounter. APPs, such as nurse practitioners or physician assistants, often practice telehealth and function either independently or under the supervision of an attending physician (Rutledge et al., 2017). As most of the training for this group will be similar to either GME or faculty, for this chapter, APPs will be categorized as such unless specified. Clinical tele-presenters, however, are a group of nonphysician or APP medical staff who also do telehealth visits. They function to "present" a patient over virtual care to another provider and are most often used within provider-to-provider consults. They can be nurses, technicians, or other staff trained in the particular type of exam. Because they also need training in physical exam, this group will be included under those being trained in this type of care (Sikka et al., 2021).

When to Train

Initially, training was set up for programs that existed and for those staffing the telehealth programs. There was a recent increased need to expand the training to UME, GME, and new programs around the country. Regardless, as telehealth has grown significantly and is being utilized in numerous ways, the education of how to do it and learning

physical exam skills should be included at every training level (Annis et al., 2020; Hollander & Carr, 2020; Ko, 2020; Rheuban, 2020; SAEM, n.d.; Snapiri et al., 2020).

Clinical Tele-Presenters

The focus of utilizing the clinical tele-presenter is helping practitioners understand the telemedicine modality, **webside manner**, and utilization of good communication with the distant-site clinician. Clinical tele-presenters typically have the medical skills to assist with the physical exam, history taking, and communication. Training can be tailored to the level of clinical experience and the telemedicine use case. For example, tele-presenters doing endocrinology tele-consults were taught how to conduct monofilament testing, something with which many ancillary clinical team members are less familiar (Wilson et al., 2020). Tailoring the training will be based on a needs assessment of the specific program.

Undergraduate Medical Education

As more programs incorporate telehealth in various clinical departments, this requires that medical students also would be exposed during their clinical rotations. At this level, provision of a general background and introduction to the basics of telehealth visits as well as virtual physical exam is necessary. As UME students learn physical exam in their preclinical years, they should be exposed to telehealth principles as they would to other types of relevant information for their future healthcare career. For example, Jefferson Health readied its UME students to return to clinical rotations in June of 2020 by creating a module on telehealth. These at-home training modules allowed the students to access the material later on as needed and provided an effective introduction to telehealth. Other programs also initiated training and education (Abraham et al., 2020; Cantone et al., 2019). In general, training should be relevant to the clinician's skill level (Waseh & Dicker, 2019).

Graduate Medical Education

Residents are already clinical and working within their respective fields, so the priority is teaching specialty-tailored telehealth. These tips are also relevant to other medical professionals in their training. One of the ways to do this is to evaluate and understand the type of telehealth physical exam necessary for that particular group; however, the understanding is that residents are still in training and require the supervision of their attendings. To this end, each of the different specialties can tailor their training for physical exam based on what is most important and relevant to their needs (Keswani et al., 2020; Papanagnou et al., 2018). The Medical College of South Carolina, for example, created a curriculum specifically geared for telehealth for GME, and other institutions will likely follow their lead (Medical University of South Carolina, n.d.).

Advanced Practice Provider Training

Depending on state laws and regulations, APPs either function independently or under a physician's license. Their training is then relevant to the type of practice and whether it needs to be supervised, and training should be thought of similarly. Training can be similarly done while in school, in training, or for program-specific implementations (Rutledge et al., 2017).

Faculty/Attending Training

Faculty or attending training relies on the physician knowing their clinical practice and needing training to tailor their knowledge to telehealth. These tips are also relevant to other practicing medical professionals. It can be hypothesized that training is easier when one understands and feels comfortable in one's in-person clinical practice. In these cases, one has only to understand the telehealth clinical environment and be able to use the same skills in that modality. The pandemic created a crucial need to convert quickly to virtual care, forcing more practitioners to try out virtual clinical medical encounters, likely with little training due to the paucity of programs (Chou et al., 2020; Hamm et al., 2020; Joshi et al., 2020a; Lau et al., 2020; Lin et al., 2020; Wittbold et al., 2020). However, simply "doing" does not always translate to understanding the extent and the limits of telehealth physical exam. For this reason, skill and experience far trump the need to understand the technology as far as doing medical encounters is concerned (Hollander & Carr, 2020; Inman, 2020).

Because there are more time constraints on faculty, the training should be high yield and efficient, and apply specifically to what trainees need to know. For the physical exam, this includes a practical guide of using the physical exam in the specific types of visits the faculty will be engaging in.

USE OF ADJUNCT DEVICES FOR EXAM

An overview of virtual physical exam is not complete without a brief mention of the current and future involvement of adjunct devices to aid in physical exam.

Some devices for home telehealth physical exam are simple: good lighting for both video and photos, good Wi-Fi connection to enable the sending of photos and use of space within a home that can aid in physical exam. One study reported discordance in pharyngeal exam when using telehealth and suggested that easily observed exam elements show high concordance, but posterior elements that are difficult to observe using consumer technology limit the utility of the pharyngitis physical examination (Akhtar et al., 2018). It should be noted that lighting can help, but there is a gap in understanding of whether photos of different skin tones may fare better or worse within the telehealth platform. This will be an important area for further analysis in the future.

Other devices are already used by patients at home, and the data from them simply have to be organized and shared to their provider; these can include weight, blood pressure, temperature, pulse oximetry, heart rate, blood glucose, and other measures for chronic disease. Most of these devices may or may not be available if the patient does not already have them. Glucometers, rapid strep swabs, and home urine tests are useful for subjective point-of-care testing for common urgent care complaints. Other devices on the market have more unique use cases, or can supply multiple vital signs within one product, and are in various stages of validation and use. Applications can aid with determining motion during family-directed abdominal exam, and electronic stethoscopes connected to Bluetooth or EKGs done with FDA-approved devices can aid in exam (Ansary et al., 2021). This is contingent on the patient having access to these tools and will likely be more utilizable in the future. A few studies noted that home devices were able to treat patients successfully at home (Notario et al., 2019), and in one study they performed better than standalone devices (McDaniel et al., 2019). While these studies are promising, there is a need for more prospective research studies to evaluate home telehealth and remote monitoring devices.

COMPONENTS OF PHYSICAL EXAM TRAINING

As all levels of learners in clinical environments will be doing similar exams overall, we can use the list of core competencies for medical education physical exam and apply those concepts to virtual care (AAMC, 2021). While much of the telehealth visit can use physical exam components, simply thinking through what could be done and tailoring it to telehealth is a vital and organized way to create education modules and training.

Training can be done in a few different ways:

- In-person training: training sessions to practice components of the virtual physical exam with standardized patients.
- Simulation training: used throughout medical education and can be adapted for students and learners to learn and practice telemedicine physical exam.
- Online learning modules: asynchronous version for at-home learning and review. This requires creating and housing these modules in an accessible portal.

There is room for validation of these types of education modules, and research steps should be taken to understand how it can be done in an effective manner.

THE PHYSICAL EXAM

The Center for Medicare and Medicaid services (CMS) has set a series of physical exam guidelines for medical encounters and this can be used as a guide for understanding what is taught and considered standard for all physicians to know. It is essential to note that these skills are taught beginning in medical school. The components of the physical exam from CMS are listed below by category (CMS, 1997). Each section will outline the standard exam and also what can be done via telehealth without adjunct devices.

Importance of History

For all virtual visits, history becomes much more important, harking back to Sir William Osler's famous adage. If, for instance, hypertension is a reason for concern and adjunct blood pressure devices are unavailable, a provider can inquire about other aspects of history to gather data, such as vision changes, numbness or tingling in extremities, or headaches. If hypotension is a concern and no devices are available, a provider can inquire about relevant history like dizziness, light-headedness, cold or clammy skin, or whether the patient's mouth feels dry or less moist than their baseline. It is important for the provider to use key aspects of the history to aid in medical decision-making when conducting an assessment remotely (Centor, 2007).

Physical Exam Guidelines per CMS

Constitutional Exam

Remote providers can rely on visualization and patients for a number of constitutional exam findings. Many of the pertinent vital signs are also obtainable.

For general appearance, it is important to note the general build of the patient and any obvious deformities or amputations. The level of alertness is a key aspect; that is, documenting whether they are awake and attentive or

---

TABLE 3.1   Constitutional Exam (CMS, 1997)

Constitutional physical exam:
- Measurement of any three of the following **seven** vital signs:
  1. sitting or standing blood pressure
  2. supine blood pressure
  3. pulse rate and regularity
  4. respiration
  5. temperature
  6. height
  7. weight (can be measured and recorded by ancillary staff)
- General appearance of patient (e.g., development, nutrition, body habitus, deformities, attention to grooming)

Telemedicine constitutional exam:
- Measurement of the following vital signs:
  1. respiratory rate
  2. pulse
- With devices or patient knowledge:
  1. blood pressure (sitting, standing, and supine)
  2. height
  3. weight
  4. temperature
- General appearance of patient (e.g., development, nutrition, body habitus, deformities, attention to grooming)

---

lethargic and confused. Make sure to note if they greet you and respond to your introduction appropriately or if they are unkempt and not responding appropriately. Noting any obvious distress—whether due to pain, respiratory distress, or other instability—also goes within this section.

For vital signs, some information will require devices that patients may or may not have at home. Those with blood pressure cuffs can take a reading or, if they are unfamiliar with the device, can be guided by the provider to properly place the cuff, position themselves, and get the most accurate blood pressure reading possible. Temperature can be gathered through an at-home thermometer if available. A provider can also ask questions regarding thermal regulation issues such as chills, sweats, flushing of the skin, and intermittent sweats.

Other vital signs can be taken under instruction. The patient can take their radial or carotid pulse and count out loud. This allows for the provider to note the rate but also whether the counts are irregular. Another option is to guide the patient to download an application on their phone to verify their heart rate, which can be done during the visit or prior if the visit was scheduled. Respiratory rate can also be counted by the provider by simply watching the patient, as with in-person encounters.

Many patients are aware of their approximate height and weight, which can be helpful in obtaining their BMI. Even if weight or height are not exact, a generalization will help to guide care and risk factor analysis. Weight changes can be significant when dealing with patients whose chronic diseases can affect weight and indicate deterioration, like congestive heart failure. The main takeaway from the constitutional section is the general appearance of the patient, their level of distress, and their overall perceived health status at that time. This aspect allows whichever provider sees the patient next to gauge if they have improved, deteriorated, or remained the same. This will ultimately influence their escalation of care if necessary.

Eye Exam

Eye exams can benefit from a picture being taken and uploaded prior to a visit, as the provider can examine and zoom in on certain aspects that may be concerning. The patient should remove any contact lenses prior to starting the exam.

With a general inspection of the eye, one can assess symmetry of the lids, sockets, and conjunctiva, and evaluate for any lid droop, injection, crusting, or exudate. The patient can be asked to retract or lift their lid based on their comfort to expose more of the palpebral conjunctiva. In our experience, this will be limited by patient willingness and comfort.

With the patient close to the camera, a flashlight or phone light can be used to examine the pupils for reaction to light and extraocular movements. Instruct the patient to shine the light into their eye and hold for a few seconds and then

remove. Using the online vision test Peek Acuity can allow for real-time visual acuity testing. One study demonstrated that the Peek Acuity smartphone test is capable of accurate and repeatable acuity measurements consistent with published data on the test-retest variability of acuities measured using five-letter-per-line retroilluminated logMAR charts (Bastawrous et al., 2015). While intraocular pressures and a slit lamp cannot yet be done as standard without home devices, an examination of the conjunctiva, lids, pupils, extraocular movements, and general vision is possible.

Ears, Nose, Mouth, and Throat Exam

The overall appearance can evaluate for scars, lesions, masses, injury, or rashes. For facial neuro deficits, the provider should look for facial symmetry, appropriate movement of the mouth, any drooling or labial flattening, ability to raise eyebrows, to smile and frown, to close the eyes tightly, to show both the lower and upper teeth, and to puff out their cheeks. One can assess the gross hearing of the patient by gauging their responsiveness to questions over the device, whether they ask for questions to be repeated, or need a hearing device at baseline.

With the video device or a still photo the provider can evaluate the lips, teeth, gums, and overall oral hygiene of the patient. Intraoral exam includes assessing the state of dentition, swelling, any gross bleeding, ulcerations, or sores and

TABLE 3.2 Eye Exam (CMS, 1997)

Eye physical exam:
- inspection of conjunctivae and lids
- examination of pupils and irises (e.g., reaction to light and accommodation, size, symmetry)
- ophthalmoscopic examination of optic discs (e.g., size, Cup to Disk (C/D) ratio, appearance) and posterior segments (e.g., vessel changes, exudates, hemorrhages)

Telemedicine eye exam:
- inspection of the conjunctiva and lids
- examination of the pupils (reaction to light and accommodation, size, symmetry)
- visual acuity via smartphone applications (limitations do exist)

TABLE 3.3 Ears, Nose, Mouth, and Throat Exam (CMS, 1997)

Ears, nose, mouth, and throat physical exam:
- external inspection of ears and nose (e.g., overall appearance, scars, lesions, masses)
- otoscopic examination of external auditory canals and tympanic membranes
- assessment of hearing (e.g., whispered voice, finger rub, tuning fork)
- inspection of nasal mucosa, septum, and turbinates
- inspection of lips, teeth, and gums
- examination of oropharynx: oral mucosa, salivary glands, hard and soft palates, tongue, tonsils, and posterior pharynx

Telemedicine ears, nose, mouth, and throat exam:
- external inspection of ears and nose (e.g., overall appearance, scars, lesions, masses)
- assessment of hearing
- inspection of nasal mucosa, external nares
- inspection of lips, teeth, and gums
- examination of oropharynx: oral mucosa, salivary glands, hard and soft palates, tongue, tonsils, and posterior pharynx

also whether there is any discoloration to the oral tissue. Using appropriate lighting and angling, one can visualize the tongue, tonsils, and posterior pharynx, looking for enlargement, exudate, or masses via visual inspection. If there are concerns with airway patency, patients can be asked to breathe with an open mouth, which could reveal concerns for an obstructive mass or stenosis (Prasad et al., 2020). Still photos are also an option. A spoon can be used as a tongue depressor to allow viewing and evaluation of the soft palate and tonsils (Prasad et al., 2020). Telemedicine exhibited poor agreement with the in-person physical examination on the primary outcome of tonsil size, but exhibited moderate agreement on coloration of the palate and cervical lymphadenopathy. Future work should better characterize the importance of the physical examination in treatment decisions for patients with sore throat and the use of telemedicine in avoiding in-person healthcare visits (Akhtar et al., 2018).

The external auditory canal and earlobe can be examined in conjunction with the patient or with family/care partner participation. The pinna and mastoid can be evaluated for tenderness and to assess whether there is bleeding or discharge at the entry of the auditory canal. Lymph node exam can also be done under provider guidance, although it may be more difficult to assess as it relies on patient/family understanding of what that means. If one is dealing with a pediatric patient, many times the parent or guardian can assist with the exam (Table 3.1).

Neck Exam

Over video the provider can note the position of the trachea, obvious masses, rashes, jugular venous distention, and the overall general appearance and symmetry of the neck. For the thyroid, visual inspection for any enlargement or masses should be performed.

With patient participation, one can assess for tender lymph nodes in the cervical or head region. A provider can guide a patient through palpation by showing them where to push and seeing whether they experience any tenderness.

While the patient is sitting, ask them to turn their head to the left, and observe the neck veins. Distension of neck veins above the clavicle while sitting is a clue to volume overload. If the patient sits next to a window, natural lighting may make observing their neck veins easier (Benziger et al., 2021). Before concluding the exam, it is important to note the range of movement in the neck and identify any deficits. Having the patient follow the provider through flexion anteriorly, posteriorly, and laterally is most constructive for the patient. Any stiffness should herald a closer exam and history and may warrant in-person evaluation.

Respiratory Exam

Currently, without a remote stethoscope, lung sounds cannot be heard and the exam requires the use of other information (Table 3.5). Overall appearance should assess for respiratory status including respiratory effort, any intercostal retractions, use of accessory muscles, diaphragmatic movement, or nasal flaring. One can assess for any audible wheezing, visible shortness of breath, cyanosis, or trouble speaking. This inspection can be done the same remotely as it would be in the office setting. The provider should make note of whether the patient can speak in full sentences or if they need to pause to catch their breath. If a provider hears a cough, it is important to note whether it is frequent, productive, or dry.

The Roth criteria (a tool for quantifying the level of breathlessness, which correlates to the level of hypoxia) have been used in the past for remote assessment of respiratory status. This tool combines maximal count reached (starting from 1 to 30 in one's native language) during a single exhalation and the time taken to reach the maximum count; the second score is called the "counting time" (Greenhalgh, 2020). The counting time would then be correlated to a level of hypoxia. Maximal counting number <10 or counting time <7 seconds

TABLE 3.4   Neck Exam (CMS, 1997)

Neck physical exam:
- examination of neck (e.g., masses, overall appearance, symmetry, tracheal position, crepitus)
- examination of thyroid (e.g., enlargement, tenderness, mass)

Telemedicine neck exam:
- examination of neck (e.g., masses, overall appearance, symmetry, tracheal position, crepitus)
- examination of thyroid (e.g., enlargement, tenderness, mass)
- assess range of motion of the neck

TABLE 3.5   Pulmonary Exam (CMS, 1997)

Respiratory physical exam:
- Assessment of respiratory effort (e.g., intercostal retractions, use of accessory muscles, diaphragmatic movement)
- Percussion of chest (e.g., dullness, flatness, hyperresonance)
- Palpation of chest (e.g., tactile fremitus)
- Auscultation of lungs (e.g., breath sounds, adventitious sounds, rubs)

Telemedicine respiratory exam:
- Assessment of respiratory effort (e.g., intercostal retractions, use of accessory muscles, diaphragmatic movement)
- Palpation of chest (e.g., reproducible pain, crepitus)

identifies patients with a room-air pulse oximetry <95% with sensitivity of 91% and 83%, respectively; maximal counting number <7 or counting time <5 seconds identifies patients with a room-air pulse oximetry <90% with sensitivity of 87% and 82%, respectively (Chorin et al., 2016).

While the criteria were published in 2016, during the COVID-19 pandemic in 2020 they were utilized much more widely due to the expansion of telehealth for screening and evaluation. The increased utility prompted a validation of the criteria, showing a strong correlation with dyspnea severity as determined by hypoxia. Although it was not intended to replace full clinical workup and diagnosis of respiratory distress, the tool was useful in risk-stratifying the severity of dyspnea that warrants further clinical evaluation at that time (Chorin et al., 2016). But the new data demonstrate that the Roth score may be normal when the patient is severely hypoxic, may be abnormal when the patient is not hypoxic, and could potentially overshadow a more holistic assessment of a patient (Greenhalgh, 2020). Given these recent COVID-19-related findings, it is no longer advised to use the Roth score to correlate with hypoxia.

Other options include the use of home pulse oximeters due to the risk of undiagnosed hypoxemia in patients feeling mild symptoms of COVID-19 (Luks & Swenson, 2020). One study used home pulse oximeters and found that patients were able to reduce ED revisits and that those needing hospitalization after having initially mild symptoms could be identified (Shah et al., 2020). Again, the use of these devices is limited by access and connectivity but can substantially help with complaints of dyspnea in acute or chronic conditions.

TABLE 3.6 Cardiovascular Exam (Greenhalgh, 2020)

Cardiovascular/chest physical exam:
- palpation of heart (e.g., location, size, thrills)
- auscultation of heart with notation of abnormal sounds and murmurs
- examination of:
  - carotid arteries (e.g., pulse amplitude, bruits)
  - abdominal aorta (e.g., size, bruits)
  - femoral arteries (e.g., pulse amplitude, bruits)
  - pedal pulses (e.g., pulse amplitude)
  - extremities for edema and/or varicosities

Telemedicine cardiovascular/chest exam:
- location of pain; if present, see if reproducible to palpation
- assess lower extremities for presence of edema
- assess pulse rate
- examine neck for jugular venous distension
- capillary refill

Cardiovascular/Chest-Exam

Currently, without a remote stethoscope, heart sounds cannot be heard and so the exam requires the use of other information. The patient can assess pain to chest wall with palpation. The patient can take their own pulse and count out loud, as noted in the constitutional exam for vital signs. This allows for the provider to note the rate and regularity. Studies demonstrating the validity of using smartphones to measure heart rate have indicated that the Android HR acquisition software embedded in a Motorola Droid smartphone provides valid measurements of heart rate while at rest and when subjects are engaging in mildly stressful motion-free perceptual motor/cognitive activities (Gregoski et al., 2012), thus demonstrating this as a possible adjunct device that might be easier for a patient to use. While the patient is sitting, ask them to turn their head to the left, and observe the neck veins. Distension of neck veins above the clavicle while sitting is a clue to volume overload. If the patient sits next to a window, natural lighting may make observing their neck veins easier (Benziger et al., 2021).

For those who have access to a digital stethoscope, this can be used for a heart and lung exam. Currently these devices use Bluetooth to link to the digital stethoscope and upload the sounds to an app, allowing them to be sent to the physician or heard synchronously (Ansary et al., 2021; Swarup & Makaryus, 2018).

A visual examination of the lower extremities can evaluate for obvious edema, rashes, mottling, or discoloration. The patient can palpate with their finger various points along the ankle, leg, and thighs, evaluating for pitting edema as well as palpating for calf tenderness. A provider can also estimate the capillary refill by coaching the patient to pinch one of their extremities for two seconds on camera, and the provider assessing the capillary refill time. Look for any discoloration or mottling in the patient's distal extremities, and ask about any noticeable temperature changes by having the patient compare with another extremity or other parts of the body.

The visual inspection of the abdomen includes looking for scars, distention, masses, asymmetry, and cutaneous changes (varicoceles or spider angiomas). For palpation, a family or care partner is necessary in order for the exam to be more akin to an in-person exam. The bystander can do the exam under the guidance of a provider who can visually inspect the technique and the patient's reaction. If no bystander is present, one can coach the patient through palpation of the abdominal quadrants; however, it is difficult to truly palpate on oneself and it is not advised for high-risk patients or complaints. The patient can bear down or tense the abdomen to elicit abdominal hernias. One option is the use of an app that evaluates the strength of palpation; however, these adjunct devices are in the validation stage (Ansary et al., 2021).

Gastrointestinal/Abdominal Exam

A validated option for the pediatric population includes having the patient jump or hop on one foot to assess right lower quadrant pain (Fig. 3.6 and 3.7). This can be used as a clinical test to demonstrate peritonism in a child complaining of right lower quadrant pain (Tzortzopoulou et al., 2019). Worth noting is that physician-guided patient self-examination via telemedicine has resulted in appropriate referral to the ED and diagnosis of appendicitis (Nachum et al., 2019). While larger validation studies need to be conducted, this demonstrates that there are ways to treat abdominal pain via telehealth.

If the patient has a complaint relevant to the rectum or perineum and they are comfortable with a video examination, a provider can guide them through the visual inspection of the exterior rectum and perineum. Still photographs taken in advance of the visit can be helpful for more detailed examination and also ensure more patient comfort if extended time is needed to visualize the area. The patient can be asked to photograph stool, allowing the examiner to inspect for the presence of blood, discoloration, or grossly viewed worms. One study noted good interreliability between virtual and in-person exam of seeing hematuria on pictures of sterile urine (Novara et al., 2020).

Breast/Chest Exam

The visual assessment of chest/breast will include any obvious masses, discoloration, or discharge from the nipple. This exam will most likely be initiated by the patient given their specific complaint. The provider should guide the patient through palpation of the breast and axilla while having them describe any masses or lumps felt and inquiring whether the area is tender upon palpation. They should also ask the patient to gently squeeze the nipple; it is important to note any discharge or bleeding.

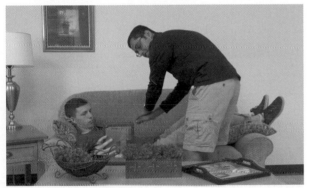

Fig. 3.6 Using a care partner to help perform palpation during an abdominal exam. (Thomas Jefferson University Telehealth Department)

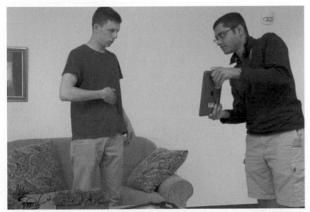

Fig. 3.7 Remotely guiding a patient through self-palpation during an abdominal exam. (Thomas Jefferson University Telehealth Department)

TABLE 3.7 Abdominal Exam (CMS, 1997)

Gastrointestinal/abdominal physical exam:
- examination of abdomen with notation of presence of masses or tenderness
- examination of liver and spleen
- examination for presence or absence of hernia
- examination (when indicated) of anus, perineum, and rectum, including sphincter tone, presence of hemorrhoids, and rectal masses
- obtain stool sample for occult blood test when indicated

Telemedicine gastrointestinal/abdominal exam:
- examination of abdomen with notation of presence of masses or tenderness
- distension or tenderness of the liver and spleen
- examination for presence or absence of hernia
- examination (when indicated) of anus and perineum, including presence of external hemorrhoids and rectal masses
- examine stool visually for gross blood, mucus, or color change

TABLE 3.8 Breast/Chest Exam (CMS, 1997)

Breast/chest physical exam:
- inspection of breasts (e.g., symmetry, nipple discharge)
- palpation of breasts and axillae (e.g., masses or lumps, tenderness)

Telemedicine breast/chest exam:
- inspection of breasts (e.g., symmetry, nipple discharge, cutaneous changes)
- palpation of breasts and axillae (e.g., masses or lumps, tenderness)

TABLE 3.9   Genitourinary Exam (Male) (CMS, 1997)

Genitourinary physical exam (male):
- examination of the scrotal contents (e.g., hydrocele, spermatocele, tenderness of cord, testicular mass)
- examination of the penis
- digital rectal examination of the prostate gland (e.g., size, symmetry, nodularity, tenderness)

Telemedicine genitourinary exam (male):
- examination of the scrotum exteriorly and via palpation (e.g., tenderness of cord, testicular mass)
- examination of the penis shaft and glans

TABLE 3.10   Genitourinary Exam (Female) (CMS, 1997)

Genitourinary physical exam (female):
- pelvic examination (with or without specimen collection for smears and cultures), including:
  - external genitalia (e.g., general appearance, hair distribution, lesions) and vagina (e.g., general appearance, estrogen effect, discharge, lesions, pelvic support, cystocele, rectocele)
  - urethra (e.g., masses, tenderness, scarring)
  - bladder (e.g., fullness, masses, tenderness)
  - cervix (e.g., general appearance, lesions, discharge)
  - uterus (e.g., size, contour, position, mobility, tenderness, consistency, descent or support)
  - adnexa/parametria (e.g., masses, tenderness, organomegaly, nodularity)
- lymphatic palpation of lymph nodes in two or more areas:
  - neck
  - axillae
  - groin
  - other

Telemedicine genitourinary exam (female):
- examination of external genitalia (e.g., general appearance, hair distribution, lesions) and vagina (e.g., general appearance, estrogen effect, discharge, exterior lesions)
- examination of urethra (e.g., masses, tenderness, scarring)
- lymphatic palpation of lymph nodes in two or more areas:
  - neck
  - axillae
  - groin
  - other

Genitourinary Exam

Start with an overall visual inspection of the penis and scrotal area, evaluating for lesions, cutaneous changes, masses, or noted swelling. Verbally guide the patient through palpation of the testicle, asking them to describe any area of tenderness or mass they may feel. Ask them to palpate the shaft of the penis and to attempt to expel any drainage in the penis, making note if any is present. At this time, it is not advisable for a digital rectal exam to be done by the patient as there is no evidence demonstrating its efficacy. If concerned about any rectal or prostate process, the patient should be advised for an in-provider assessment.

For the female genitourinary exam, it is important to survey the external urethra, vagina, and pubic region, noting any masses, lesions, cutaneous changes, scarring, unusual hair patterns, obvious discharge, or bruising. Guide the patient through palpation of the regional lymph nodes, noting any tenderness. During this exam the patient will be exposed, so pay prompt attention to any area of concern for the patient. This allows the provider to address it early on in the exam and minimize the time the patient is exposed or uncomfortable. A full intravaginal exam is not possible so, depending on complaint, risk factors and screening patients should be evaluated for in-person exam.

Musculoskeletal Exam

Many aspects of the musculoskeletal exam can be conducted remotely (Fig. 3.8). Based on the area of concern, the visual inspection can note misalignment, asymmetry, masses, defects, joint effusion, cyanosis, edema, wounds, ischemic changes, petechiae or cutaneous changes, including erythema, tracking, or exterior signs of infection.

One can also use patient participation to assess range of motion and what elicits pain. One can assess the gait of the patient, noticing if they stand with or without the use of arms to push off of a chair, whether the gait is broad or narrow, or if they have any pain with movement (Wahezi et al., 2020).

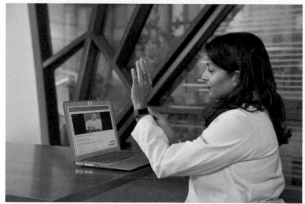

Fig. 3.8 Dr. Aditi U. Joshi guiding a patient remotely through a wrist exam. (Thomas Jefferson University Photography Services)

TABLE 3.11 Notes on Sensitive Exams

The breast exam and genitourinary exams of males and females are considered sensitive exams. A valid concern is how to navigate this over telehealth and whether it is safe.

Generally, it is essential to evaluate patient comfort, and any hint or feeling of exposure should prompt an in-person evaluation. The patient should be reassured that the visit is a medical encounter and secure; however, any doubt should warrant sending the patient in for exam.

If the patient is comfortable, the options include securely uploading a picture to the exam session, which would be part of the medical record and decrease live exposure for the patient. There will be times when this may not be enough information and a further exam is needed. For these exams, the provider can ask a chaperone to be present, as would be the case in any office setting. The chaperone should ideally be someone from the provider network rather than a family member, although the latter may be the only person available. The patient should understand and consent to the exam and chaperone available.

We also only advise this if the patient is comfortable with a sensitive exam via telehealth. One should apply the same etiquette and guidelines as if they were treating a patient in person.

TABLE 3.12 Ottawa Ankle and Foot Rules (Stiell, 1996)

An ankle x-ray series is only required if there is:
- pain in the malleolar zone
- bone tenderness at the posterior edge or tip of the lateral malleolus
- bone tenderness at the posterior edge or tip of the medial malleolus
- an inability to bear weight both immediately and when walking for four steps

A foot x-ray series is only rrequired if there is:
- any pain in the midfoot zone and bone tenderness at the base of the fifth metatarsal or bone tenderness at the navicular bone
- an inability to bear weight both immediately and when walking for four steps

The Ottawa ankle rule project demonstrated that more than 95% of patients with ankle injuries had radiographic examinations, but that 85% of the films showed no fractures. Due to this, a group of Ottawa emergency physicians developed two rules to identify clinically important

TABLE 3.13 Skin Exam (CMS, 1997)

Skin physical exam:
- inspection of skin and subcutaneous tissue (e.g., rashes, lesions, ulcers)
- palpation of skin and subcutaneous tissue (e.g., induration, subcutaneous nodules, tightening

Telemedicine skin exam:
- inspection of skin and subcutaneous tissue (e.g., rashes, lesions, ulcers)
- palpation of skin and subcutaneous tissue by the patient (e.g., induration, subcutaneous nodules, tightening, pain, temperature changes)

fractures of the malleoli and the midfoot. Use of these rules reduced radiographic examinations by 28% for the ankle and 14% for the foot and the rules are widely used in acute care medicine (Stiell, 1996). Studies have been done using the Ottawa ankle rules via telemedicine for suspected ankle injuries and showing their effectiveness (Sikka, n.d.).

Skin Exam

The skin exam seems an obvious one to tailor to telehealth; however, poor lighting or reduced-quality pictures can affect the caliber of the exam. It is beneficial to use multiple photographs from the patient which will allow the provider to assess the skin under different lighting, and to zoom in and out of the photo to gather more information. One can have the patient show the area of concern under different lighting, including lamp light, near a window, or even outside in sunlight. The inspection of the skin will look for rashes, lesions, and ulcers, along with any subcutaneous nodules or tightening. One can also notice any cracking, fissures, mottling, petechiae, cyanosis, diaphoresis, discharge, erythema, or strongly demarcated areas of the skin. The patient would be involved to evaluate the skin for temperature, injury to the affected area, pain upon palpation, and blanching.

Studies on the effectiveness and quality of teledermatology show promise that this can be done effectively, at least for certain dermatological complaints (Bashshur et al., 2015; Bastola et al., 2021; Finnane et al., 2017). A 2020 meta-analysis noted that there are varying results when studies investigate the diagnostic concordance of telehealth vs in-person visits for dermatology; however, there are some tips to aid the practitioner. To optimize visits, studies recommend using pictures instead of live video, well-lit rooms, and using cards/rulers as measuring devices (Bastola et al., 2021).

Neurologic Exam

Initial appearance and inspection can include gait, movement, assessing orientation, speech and memory, and looking for any signs of facial droop (Fig. 3.9). While home

TABLE 3.14   Neurologic Exam (CMS, 1997)

Neurologic physical exam:

- test cranial nerves with notation of any deficits
- test coordination (e.g., finger/nose, heel/knee/shin, rapid alternating movements in the upper and lower extremities, evaluation of fine motor coordination in young children)
- examination of deep tendon reflexes and/or nerve stretch test with notation of pathological reflexes (e.g., Babinski)
- examination of sensation (e.g., by touch, pin, vibration, proprioception)
- brief assessment of mental status including orientation to time, place and person, mood and affect (e.g., depression, anxiety, agitation)

Telemedicine neurologic exam:

- test cranial nerves with notation of any deficits
- test coordination (e.g., finger/nose, heel/knee/shin, rapid alternating movements in the upper and lower extremities, evaluation of fine motor coordination in young children)
- examination of deep tendon reflexes with patient participation
- examination of sensation (e.g., by touch, pin)
- brief assessment of mental status including orientation to time, place and person, mood and affect (e.g., depression, anxiety, agitation)

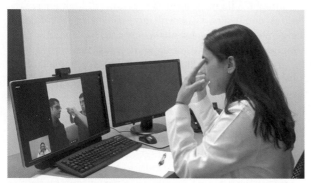

Fig. 3.9 Dr. Kristin Rising conducting a neurological assessment remotely with the aid of a care partner. (Thomas Jefferson University Telehealth Department)

visits will not have the advantage of a medical trained professional, parts of the neuro exam can still be done with either patient or family/care partner participation. They can help assess cranial nerves and ask the patient to reference specific changes in sensation using objects commonly found in the home; for example, a pen and a tissue. The patient can be instructed to outline any dermatomal distribution of any pain or altered sensation. Gross motor deficits are elicited during the exam with the patient's participation of movement and gait.

Tele-stroke is one of the longest-running use cases of telehealth, in which telemedicine is used for stroke assessment between hub and spoke centers (LaMonte et al., 2003). In one study, telemedicine examination was more sensitive in detecting abnormalities than face-to-face examination for all the neurologic tests studied and more specific for all but one, plantar responses (Craig et al., 1999). During the COVID-19 pandemic, rapid adoption of virtual medicine was critical to provide ongoing and timely neurological care (Al Hussona et al., 2020). Remote assessment was a reliable way to decrease exposure to the providers while still allowing for proper care and triage. We recognize that despite these promising studies, tele-stroke has two providers (or a provider and tele-presenter), both parties who are trained in the exam, which is not the case for at-home care.

Mental and behavioral health assessment over telehealth has a number of practitioners and there are noted benefits to improve access to care. A review of past research showed telepsychiatry is effectual and increases healthcare accessibility (Stiens, 2019). Since there is little actual physical contact between patient and provider for this exam, it uses and relies more heavily on webside manner and connecting effectively. The concerns have mostly been about connecting similarly with patients over video rather than through the components of the psychiatric exam; the issue of webside manner is discussed in Chapter 11.

In short, the provider can visually inspect a patient's affect, demeanor, and speech over telehealth. They can do their mental status exam, assess for pressured speech, mood liability, suicidal or homicidal ideation and thoughts, and conduct a complete psychiatric exam. The evidence to date is highly suggestive that telepsychiatry is comparable to face-to-face care on several aspects of what is traditionally considered effectiveness (Chakrabarti, 2015; Kerst et al., 2020; Torniainen-Holm et al., 2016; Zhou et al., 2020).

DISCUSSION

The components of the physical exam taught to learners currently do not specifically focus on telehealth, so this guide is aimed to give an understanding of practical tips based on experience and current research. This list is not exhaustive; it does not include applications and devices, or home care workers and others who may be trained to help, and longtime practitioners may have other tips for their exam not covered here. In the future, the goal is to be able to add these telehealth virtual exam components as a

TABLE 3.15   Top Tips for Improved Virtual Physical Exam Encounters

✓ Before looking in the mouth/throat, have the patient place a finger over the camera lens to warm it up so it won't fog from their warm breath when the exam takes place.

✓ When assessing masses, it helps to guide patients using everyday references they are accustomed to. For example, does it feel soft like a grape or hard like an almond? This will allow the patient to describe things they are familiar with and aid the provider with information they themselves cannot obtain.

✓ When obtaining the respiratory rate, if video is unavailable a provider can instruct the patient to stand in front of a mirror and count how many times their breath fogs up the mirror while the provider times them.

✓ Guide the patient with objects like a blunt pen, a soft Q-tip, or a piece of fabric for the sensation exam. Making them feel comfortable by using objects they have for the exam will likely encourage participation.

✓ A spoon (something all patients have at home) can be used as a tongue depressor to evaluate and view the soft palate and tonsils.

✓ When assessing a pediatric patient, ask the parent or guardian to assist with the exam, explaining what you are looking for and using them as your proxy.

✓ For patients with congestive heart failure or volume overload concerns, ask them to sit next to a window; natural lighting may make observing the neck veins easier.

✓ When assessing rashes or skin concerns, ask the patient to show the area of concern under different lighting, including lamp light, near a window, or even outside in sunlight.

✓ The patient can take their radial or carotid pulse and count out loud to you. This allows you to note the rate but also whether the counts are irregular.

competency in medical education, allowing for an expansion of our scope of practice in any virtual setting.

Training, understanding, and adding to virtual physical exam has the potential to improve care in the future. The shift in technology-driven remote care is here to stay and, with the increased access to care and convenience it provides, it will only gain more popularity among clinicians and patients. We have sought to determine how the exam is being used, the training currently done, and an outline of the current standardized physical exam and how it can be (and is being) tailored to telehealth. There are many advantages to understanding how to do basic physical exam components virtually; it can increase use cases and provider and patient comfort, decrease readmissions, and allow for home health expansion.

However, there are needed improvements and gaps in what we know and what is currently available to use. While this guide includes practical how-to tips and some of these have been researched in the literature, many of the utilizations require standardization and validation. This includes using components of physical exam and whether it is reliable for the patient or family member to do it themselves. Research is also required on interrater reliability between two providers; however, there is a barrier in creating these studies as they would require patients to be seen twice—virtually and in person—so they would need a prospective study design or to be done in an environment where both may be available, such as a clinic or emergency department.

While the gaps in research and validated educational modules remain, the expansion of telehealth has increased home-based healthcare as well as inter- and intrahospital virtual care. This requires more discussion and thoughtful engagement of what physical exam components or training are going to be necessary, which will be driven by standardized clinical criteria with validated research and case outcome measures.

CONCLUSION

Virtual physical exam is a necessary and utilizable part of the current and future healthcare system. It was thrust into the mainstream of healthcare for both providers and patients during the COVID-19 pandemic. Many institutions and healthcare systems adapted quickly to a field still in its infancy. Over the coming years, many changes and continued adaptations will be brought to the forefront. The goal of creating training, research, and practical tips for future providers and care partners will be necessary as they will all be part of the future home healthcare team.

REFERENCES

AAMC. (2021). *Telehealth competencies across the learning continuum. AAMC New and Emerging Areas in Medicine Series.* Washington, DC: AAMC.

Abraham, H. N., Opara, I. N., Dwaihy, R. L., et al. (2020). Engaging third-year medical students on their internal medicine clerkship in telehealth during COVID-19. *Cureus, 12*(6), e8791. https://doi.org/10.7759/cureus.8791

Akhtar, M., Van Heukelom, P. G., Ahmed, A., et al. (2018). Telemedicine physical examination utilizing a consumer device demonstrates poor concordance with in-person physical examination in emergency department patients with sore throat: A prospective blinded study. *Telemedicine Journal and e-Health*, *24*(10), 790–796. https://doi.org/10.1089/tmj.2017.0240

Al Hussona, M., Maher, M., Chan, D., et al. (2020). The virtual neurologic exam: Instructional videos and guidance for the COVID-19 Era. *The Canadian Journal of Neurological Sciences. Le Journal Canadien Des Sciences Neurologiques*, *47*(5), 598–603. https://doi.org/10.1017/cjn.2020.96

Annis, T., Pleasants, S., Hultman, G., et al. (2020). Rapid implementation of a COVID-19 remote patient monitoring program. *Journal of the American Medical Informatics Association: JAMIA*, *27*(8), 1326–1330. https://doi.org/10.1093/jamia/ocaa097

Ansary, A. M., Martinez, J. N., & Scott, J. D. (2021). The virtual physical exam in the 21st century. *Journal of Telemedicine and Telecare*, *27*(6), 382–392. https://doi.org/10.1177/1357633X19878330

Bashshur, R. L., Shannon, G. W., Tejasvi, T., et al. (2015). The empirical foundations of teledermatology: A review of the research evidence. *Telemedicine Journal and e-Health*, *21*(12), 953–979. https://doi.org/10.1089/tmj.2015.0146

Bastawrous, A., Rono, H. K., Livingstone, I. A. T., et al. (2015). Development and validation of a smartphone-based visual acuity test (peek acuity) for clinical practice and community-based fieldwork. *JAMA Ophthalmology*, *133*(8), 930–937. https://doi.org/10.1001/jamaophthalmol.2015.1468

Bastola, M., Locatis, C., & Fontelo, P. (2021). Diagnostic reliability of in-person versus remote dermatology: A meta-analysis. *Telemedicine Journal and e-Health*, *27*(3), 247–250. https://doi.org/10.1089/tmj.2020.0043

Benziger, C. P., Huffman, M. D., Sweis, R. N., et al. (2021). The telehealth ten: A guide for a patient-assisted virtual physical examination. *The American Journal of Medicine*, *134*(1), 48–51. https://doi.org/10.1016/j.amjmed.2020.06.015

Bonney, A., Knight-Billington, P., Mullan, J., et al. (2015). The telehealth skills, training, and implementation project: An evaluation protocol. *JMIR Research Protocols*, *4*(1), e2. https://doi.org/10.2196/resprot.3613

Brecthel, L., Gainey, J., Penwell, A., et al. (2018). Predictors of thrombolysis in the telestroke and non telestroke settings for hypertensive acute ischemic stroke patients. *BMC Neurology*, *18*(1), 215. https://doi.org/10.1186/s12883-018-1204-3

Cantone, R. E., Palmer, R., Dodson, L. G., et al. (2019). Insomnia telemedicine OSCE (TeleOSCE): A simulated standardized patient video-visit case for clerkship students. *MedEdPORTAL : The Journal of Teaching and Learning Resources*, *15*, 10867. https://doi.org/10.15766/mep_2374-8265.10867

Cao, Y., Li, Q., Chen, J., et al. (2020, April). Hospital emergency management plan during the COVID-19 epidemic. *Academic Emergency Medicine*, *27*, 309–311. https://doi.org/10.1111/acem.13951

Carvalho, V. S. J., Picanço, M. R., Volschan, A., et al. (2019). Impact of simulation training on a telestroke network.

International Journal of Stroke, *14*(5), 500–507. https://doi.org/10.1177/1747493018791030

CDC. (2020). *Using telehealth to expand access to essential health services during the COVID-19 pandemic.* www.cdc.gov/coronavirus/2019-ncov/hcp/telehealth.html. [Accessed 31 October 2021].

Centor, R. M. (2007). To be a great physician, you must understand the whole story. *MedGenMed: Medscape General Medicine*, *9*(1), 59.

Chaffin, H. M., Nakagawa, K., & Koenig, M. A. (2019). Impact of statewide telestroke network on acute stroke treatment in Hawai'i. *Hawai'i Journal of Health & Social Welfare*, *78*(9), 280–286.

Chakrabarti, S. (2015). Usefulness of telepsychiatry: A critical evaluation of videoconferencing-based approaches. *World Journal of Psychiatry*, *5*(3), 286–304. https://doi.org/10.5498/wjp.v5.i3.286

Chauhan, V., Galwankar, S., Arquilla, B., et al. (2020). Novel coronavirus (COVID-19): Leveraging telemedicine to optimize care while minimizing exposures and viral transmission. *Journal of Emergencies Trauma and Shock*, *13*(1), 20–24. https://doi.org/10.4103/JETS.JETS_32_20

Chen, T.-Y., Lai, H.-W., Hou, I.-L., et al. (2020). Buffer areas in emergency department to handle potential COVID-19 community infection in Taiwan. *Travel Medicine and Infectious Disease*, *36*, 101635. https://doi.org/10.1016/j.tmaid.2020.101635

Chorin, E., Padegimas, A., Havakuk, O., et al. (2016). Assessment of respiratory distress by the Roth score. *Clinical Cardiology*, *39*(11), 636–639. https://doi.org/10.1002/clc.22586

Chou, E., Hsieh, Y.-L., Wolfshohl, J., et al. (2020). Onsite telemedicine strategy for coronavirus (COVID-19) screening to limit exposure in ED. *Emergency Medicine Journal : Engineering Management Journal*, *37*(6), 335–337. https://doi.org/10.1136/emermed-2020-209645

CMS. (1997). *1997 Documentation guidelines for evaluation and management services.* https://www.cms.gov/outreach-and-education/medicare-learning-network-mln/mlnedwebguide/downloads/97docguidelines.pdf.

Craig, J. J., McConville, J. P., Patterson, V. H., et al. (1999). Neurological examination is possible using telemedicine. *Journal of Telemedicine and Telecare*, *5*(3), 177–181. https://doi.org/10.1258/1357633991933594

Davis, C. B., Marzec, L. N., Blea, Z., et al. (2019). Antibiotic prescribing patterns for sinusitis within a direct-to-consumer virtual urgent care. *Telemedicine Journal and e-Health*, *25*(6), 519–522. https://doi.org/10.1089/tmj.2018.0100

DeJong, C., Lucey, C. R., & Dudley, R. A. (2015). Incorporating a new technology while doing no harm, virtually. *JAMA*, *314*(22), 2351–2352. https://doi.org/10.1001/jama.2015.13572

Demaerschalk, B. M., Berg, J., Chong, B. W., et al. (2017). American telemedicine Association: Telestroke guidelines. *Telemedicine Journal and e-Health*, *23*(5), 376–389. https://doi.org/10.1089/tmj.2017.0006

Edirippulige, S., & Armfield, N. R. (2017). Education and training to support the use of clinical telehealth: A review of the literature. *Journal of Telemedicine and Telecare*, *23*(2), 273–282. https://doi.org/10.1177/1357633X16632968

Finnane, A., Dallest, K., Janda, M., et al. (2017). Teledermatology for the diagnosis and management of skin cancer: A systematic review. *JAMA Dermatology, 153*(3), 319–327. https://doi.org/10.1001/jamadermatol.2016.4361

Flodgren, G., Rachas, A., Farmer, A. J., et al. (2015). Interactive telemedicine: Effects on professional practice and health care outcomes. *Cochrane Database of Systematic Reviews, 2015*(9), CD002098. https://doi.org/10.1002/14651858. CD002098.pub2.

Grange, E. S., Neil, E. J., Stoffel, M., et al. (2020). Responding to COVID-19: The UW medicine information technology services experience. *Applied Clinical Informatics, 11*(2), 265–275. https://doi.org/10.1055/s-0040-1709715

Greenhalgh, T. (2020, April 2). *Question: Should the Roth score be used in the remote assessment of patients with possible COVID-19? Answer: No. Centre for Evidence-Based Medicine.* www.cebm.net/covid-19/roth-score-not-recommended-to-assess-breathlessness-over-the-phone/. [Accessed 31 October 2021].

Gregoski, M. J., Mueller, M., Vertegel, A., et al. (2012). Development and validation of a smartphone heart rate acquisition application for health promotion and wellness telehealth applications. *International Journal of Telemedicine and Applications, 2012*, 696324. https://doi.org/10.1155/2012/696324

Halpren-Ruder, D., Chang, A. M., Hollander, J. E., et al. (2019). Quality assurance in telehealth: Adherence to evidence-based indicators. *Telemedicine Journal and e-Health, 25*(7), 599–603. https://doi.org/10.1089/tmj.2018.0149

Hamm, J. M., Greene, C., Sweeney, M., et al. (2020). Telemedicine in the emergency department in the era of COVID-19: Front-line experiences from 2 institutions. *Journal of the American College of Emergency Physicians Open, 1*(6), 1630–1636. https://doi.org/10.1002/emp2.12204

Handschu, R., Littmann, R., Reulbach, U., et al. (2003). Telemedicine in emergency evaluation of acute stroke: Interrater agreement in remote video examination with a novel multimedia system. *Stroke, 34*(12), 2842–2846. https://doi.org/10.1161/01.STR.0000102043.70312.E9

Hart, D., Bond, W., Siegelman, J. N., et al. (2018). Simulation for assessment of milestones in emergency medicine residents. *Academic Emergency Medicine, 25*(2), 205–220. https://doi.org/10.1111/acem.13296

Hemingway, J. F., Singh, N., & Starnes, B. W. (2020). Emerging practice patterns in vascular surgery during the COVID-19 pandemic. *Journal of Vascular Surgery, 72*, 396–402. https://doi.org/10.1016/j.jvs.2020.04.492

Hollander, J. E., & Carr, B. G. (2020). Virtually perfect? Telemedicine for Covid-19. *New England Journal of Medicine, 382*(18), 1679–1681. https://doi.org/10.1056/NEJMp2003539

Hron, J. D., Parsons, C. R., Williams, L. A., et al. (2020). Rapid implementation of an inpatient telehealth program during the COVID-19 pandemic. *Applied Clinical Informatics, 11*(3), 452–459. https://doi.org/10.1055/s-0040-1713635

Inman, K. (2020, April 14). Telemedicine training proves vital during COVID-19 crisis, increasing access to care. *Cornell Chronicle.* https://news.cornell.edu/stories/2020/04/telemedicine-training-proves-vital-during-covid-19-crisis. [Accessed 31 October 2021]

Izzo, J. A., Watson, J., Bhat, R., et al. (2018). Diagnostic accuracy of a rapid telemedicine encounter in the emergency department. *The American Journal of Emergency Medicine, 36*(11), 2061–2063. https://doi.org/10.1016/j.ajem.2018.08.022

Jee, M., Khamoudes, D., Brennan, A. M., et al. (2020). COVID-19 outbreak response for an emergency department using in situ simulation. *Cureus, 12*(4), e7876. https://doi.org/10.7759/cureus.7876

Johnson, K. M., Dumkow, L. E., Burns, K. W., et al. (2019). Comparison of diagnosis and prescribing practices between virtual visits and office visits for adults diagnosed with sinusitis within a primary care network. *Open Forum Infectious Diseases, 6*(9), ofz393. https://doi.org/10.1093/ofid/ofz393

Jonas, C. E., Durning, S. J., Zebrowski, C., et al. (2019). An interdisciplinary, multi-institution telehealth course for third-year medical students. *Academic Medicine, 94*(6), 833–837. https://doi.org/10.1097/ACM.0000000000002701

Joshi, A. U., Lewiss, R. E., Aini, M., et al. (2020a). Solving community SARS-CoV-2 testing with telehealth: Development and implementation for screening, evaluation and testing. *JMIR MHealth and UHealth, 8*(10), e20419. https://doi.org/10.2196/20419

Joshi, A. U., Randolph, F. T., Chang, A. M., et al. (2020b). Impact of emergency department tele-intake on left without being seen and throughput metrics. *Academic Emergency Medicine, 27*(2), 139–147. https://doi.org/10.1111/accm.13890

Kerst, A., Zielasek, J., & Gaebel, W. (2020). Smartphone applications for depression: a systematic literature review and a survey of health care professionals' attitudes towards their use in clinical practice. *European Archives of Psychiatry and Clinical Neuroscience, 270*(2), 139–152. https://doi.org/10.1007/s00406-018-0974-3

Keswani, A., Brooks, J. P., & Khoury, P. (2020). The future of telehealth in allergy and immunology training. *Journal of Allergy and Clinical Immunology: In Practice, 8*(7), 2135–2141. https://doi.org/10.1016/j.jaip.2020.05.009

Ko, K. J. (2020). Launching an emergency department telehealth program during COVID-19. *Journal of Geriatric Emergency Medicine.* https://gedcollaborative.com/jgem/vol1-is7-launching-an-ed-telehealth-program-during-covid-19-real-world-implementations-for-older-adults/. [Accessed 29 October 2021].

LaMonte, M. P., Bahouth, M. N., Hu, P., et al. (2003). Telemedicine for acute stroke: Triumphs and pitfalls. *Stroke, 34*(3), 725–728. https://doi.org/10.1161/01.STR.0000056945.36583.37

Lau, J., Knudsen, J., Jackson, H., et al. (2020). Staying connected in the COVID-19 pandemic: Telehealth at the largest safety-net system in the United States. *Health Affairs, 39*(8), 1437–1442. https://doi.org/10.1377/hlthaff.2020.00903

LCME. (2011). Functions and structure of a standards for accreditation of medical education programs leading to the M. D. degree. Functions and structure of a medical school. *Medical Education.*

Lin, C.-H., Tseng, W.-P., Wu, J.-L., et al. (2020). A double triage and telemedicine protocol to optimize infection control in an emergency department in Taiwan during the

COVID-19 pandemic: Retrospective feasibility study. *Journal of Medical Internet Research*, 22(6), e20586. https://doi.org/10.2196/20586

Luks, A. M., & Swenson, E. R. (2020). Pulse oximetry for monitoring patients with COVID-19 at home. Potential pitfalls and practical guidance. *Annals of the American Thoracic Society*, 17(9), 1040–1046. https://doi.org/10.1513/AnnalsATS.202005-418FR

McDaniel, N. L., Novicoff, W., Gunnell, B., et al. (2019). Comparison of a novel handheld telehealth device with stand-alone examination tools in a clinic setting. *Telemedicine Journal and e-Health*, 25(12), 1225–1230. https://doi.org/10.1089/tmj.2018.0214

Medical University of South Carolina. (n.d.). *Telehealth for the Resident Physician*.

Moore, M. A., Coffman, M., Jetty, A., et al. (2017). Family physicians report considerable interest in, but limited use of, telehealth services. *The Journal of the American Board of Family Medicine: JABFM*, 30(3), 320–330. https://doi.org/10.3122/jabfm.2017.03.160201

Nachum, S., Stern, M. E., Greenwald, P. W., et al. (2019). Use of physician-guided patient self-examination to diagnose appendicitis: A telemedicine case report. *Telemedicine Journal and e-Health*, 25(8), 769–771. https://doi.org/10.1089/tmj.2018.0115

National Quality Forum. (2017). *Creating a framework to support measure development for telehealth, (June), 1–53*. https://doi.org/10.1007/s00442-013-2847-9

Notario, P. M., Gentile, E., Amidon, M., et al. (2019). Home-based telemedicine for children with medical complexity. *Telemedicine Journal and e-Health*, 25(11), 1123–1132. https://doi.org/10.1089/tmj.2018.0186

Novara, G., Checcucci, E., Crestani, A., et al. (2020). Telehealth in urology: A systematic review of the literature. How much can telemedicine be useful during and after the COVID-19 pandemic? *European Urology*, 78(6), 786–811. https://doi.org/10.1016/j.eururo.2020.06.025

Ochiai, H., Ohta, H., Kanemaru, K., et al. (2020). Implementation of a telestroke system for general physicians without a nearby stroke center to shorten the time to intravenous thrombolysis for acute cerebral infarction. *Acute Medicine & Surgery*, 7(1), e551. https://doi.org/10.1002/ams2.551

O'Connor, M., Asdornwised, U., Dempsey, M. L., et al. (2016). Using telehealth to reduce all-cause 30-day hospital readmissions among heart failure patients receiving skilled home health services. *Applied Clinical Informatics*, 7(2), 238–247. https://doi.org/10.4338/ACI-2015-11-SOA-0157

Papanagnou, D., Stone, D., Chandra, S., et al. (2018). Integrating telehealth emergency department follow-up visits into residency training. *Cureus*, 10(4), e2433. https://doi.org/10.7759/cureus.2433

Pathipati, A. S., Azad, T. D., & Jethwani, K. (2016). Telemedical education: Training digital natives in telemedicine. *Journal of Medical Internet Research*, 18(7), e193. https://doi.org/10.2196/jmir.5534

Powell, R. E., Stone, D., & Hollander, J. E. (2018). Patient and health system experience with implementation of an enterprise-wide telehealth scheduled video visit program: Mixed-methods study. *JMIR Medical Informatics*, 6(1), e10. https://doi.org/10.2196/medinform.8479

Prasad, A., Brewster, R., Newman, J. G., et al. (2020). Optimizing your telemedicine visit during the COVID-19 pandemic: Practice guidelines for patients with head and neck cancer. *Head & Neck*, 42(6), 1317–1321. https://doi.org/10.1002/hed.26197

Rastogi, R., Martinez, K. A., Gupta, N., et al. (2020). Management of urinary tract infections in direct to consumer telemedicine. *Journal of General Internal Medicine*, 35(3), 643–648. https://doi.org/10.1007/s11606-019-05415-7

Redford, G. (2020). *Delivering more care remotely will be critical as COVID-19 races through communities*. www.aamc.org/news-insights/delivering-more-care-remotely-will-be-critical-covid-19-races-through-communities. [Accessed 31 October 2021].

Reed, M. E., Huang, J., Graetz, I., et al. (2020). Patient characteristics associated with choosing a telemedicine visit vs office visit with the same primary care clinicians. *JAMA Network Open*, 3(6), e205873. https://doi.org/10.1001/jamanetworkopen.2020.5873

Reid, M. W., Krishnan, S., Berget, C., et al. (2018). CoYoT1 clinic: Home telemedicine increases young adult engagement in diabetes care. *Diabetes Technology & Therapeutics*, 20(5), 370–379. https://doi.org/10.1089/dia.2017.0450

Rheuban, K. (2020, June 26). *FCC Grant to Expand UVA Health's COVID-19 Telehealth Care*. https://newsroom.uvahealth.com/2020/06/26/fcc-grant-expands-uva-health-covid-19-telehealth-care/. [Accessed 31 October 2021].

Rutledge, C. M., Kott, K., Schweickert, P. A., et al. (2017). Telehealth and eHealth in nurse practitioner training: Current perspectives. *Advances in Medical Education and Practice*, 8, 399–409. https://doi.org/10.2147/AMEP.S116071

Shah, S., Majmudar, K., Stein, A., et al. (2020). Novel use of home pulse oximetry monitoring in COVID-19 patients discharged from the emergency department identifies need for hospitalization. *Academic Emergency Medicine*, 27(8), 681–692. https://doi.org/10.1111/acem.14053

Shi, Z., Mehrotra, A., Gidengil, C. A., et al. (2018). Quality of care for acute respiratory infections during direct-to-consumer telemedicine visits for adults. *Health Affairs*, 37(12), 2014–2023. https://doi.org/10.1377/hlthaff.2018.05091

Shigekawa, E., Fix, M., Corbett, G., et al. (2018). The current state of telehealth evidence: A rapid review. *Health Affairs*, 37(12), 1975–1982. https://doi.org/10.1377/hlthaff.2018.05132

Sikka, N. (n.d.). *Leveraging telehealth to expand access to high-quality care*.

Sikka, N., Gross, H., Joshi, A. U., et al. (2021). Defining emergency telehealth. *Journal of Telemedicine and Telecare*, 27(8), 527–530. https://doi.org/10.1177/1357633X19891653

Slovensky, D. J., Malvey, D. M., & Neigel, A. R. (2017). A model for mHealth skills training for clinicians: Meeting the future now. *mHealth*, 3, 24. https://doi.org/10.21037/mhealth.2017.05.03

Snapiri, O., Rosenberg Danziger, C., Krause, I., et al. (2020). Delayed diagnosis of paediatric appendicitis during the COVID-19 pandemic. *Acta Paediatrica*, *109*(8), 1672–1676. https://doi.org/10.1111/apa.15376

Spina, S., Marrazzo, F., Migliari, M., et al. (2020). The response of Milan's emergency medical system to the COVID-19 outbreak in Italy. *Lancet (London, England)*, *395*, e49–e50. https://doi.org/10.1016/S0140-6736(20)30493-1

Stanford University. (2020). *How to administer a virtual physical exam.*

Stiell, I. (1996). Ottawa ankle rules. *Canadian Family Physician Medecin de Famille Canadien*, *42*, 478–480. https://doi.org/10.7748/en.6.8.5.s10

Stiens, L. (2019). *Uses, benefits, and future directions of telepsychiatry.*

Swarup, S., & Makaryus, A. N. (2018). Digital stethoscope: Technology update. *Medical Devices (Auckland, N.Z.)*, *11*, 29–36. https://doi.org/10.2147/MDER.S135882

SAEM. (n.d.). *Telehealth in EM during the COVID crisis: Lessons learned.* SAEM.

Torniainen-Holm, M., Pankakoski, M., Lehto, T., et al. (2016). The effectiveness of email-based exercises in promoting psychological wellbeing and healthy lifestyle: A two-year follow-up study. *BMC Psychology*, *4*(1), 21. https://doi.org/10.1186/s40359-016-0125-4

Turer, R. W., Jones, I., Rosenbloom, S. T., et al. (2020). Electronic personal protective equipment: A strategy to protect emergency department providers in the age of COVID-19. *Journal of the American Medical Informatics Association: JAMIA*, *27*(6), 967–971. https://doi.org/10.1093/jamia/ocaa048

Tzortzopoulou, A. K., Giamarelou, P., Tsolia, M., et al. (2019). The Jumping Up (J-Up) test: Making the diagnosis of acute appendicitis easier in children. *Global Pediatric Health*, *6*. 2333794X19884824. https://doi.org/10.1177/2333794X19884824

Uscher-Pines, L., Mulcahy, A., Cowling, D., et al. (2016). Access and quality of care in direct-to-consumer telemedicine.

Telemedicine Journal and e-Health, *22*(4), 282–287. https://doi.org/10.1089/tmj.2015.0079

Wahezi, S. E., Duarte, R. A., Yerra, S., et al. (2020). Telemedicine during COVID-19 and beyond: A practical guide and best practices multidisciplinary approach for the orthopedic and neurologic pain physical examination. *Pain Physician*, *23*(4S), S205–S238.

Waseh, S., & Dicker, A. P. (2019). Telemedicine training in undergraduate medical education: Mixed-methods review. *JMIR Medical Education*, *5*(1), e12515. https://doi.org/10.2196/12515

Wennmann, D. O., Dlugos, C. P., Hofschröer, A., et al. (2020). [Handling of COVID-19 in the emergency department: Field report of the emergency ward of the University hospital Münster]. *Medizinische Klinik - Intensivmedizin und Notfallmedizin*, *115*(5), 380–387. https://doi.org/10.1007/s00063-020-00693-0

Whiteside, T., Kane, E., Aljohani, B., et al. (2020). Redesigning emergency department operations amidst a viral pandemic. *The American Journal of Emergency Medicine*, *38*(7), 1448–1453. https://doi.org/10.1016/j.ajem.2020.04.032

Wilson, A. M., Jamal, N. I., Cheng, E. M., et al. (2020). Teleneurology clinics for polyneuropathy: A pilot study. *Journal of Neurology*, *267*(2), 479–490. https://doi.org/10.1007/s00415-019-09553-0

Wittbold, K. A., Baugh, J. J., Yun, B. J., et al. (2020, December). iPad deployment for virtual evaluation in the emergency department during the COVID-19 pandemic. *The American Journal of Emergency Medicine*, *38*, 2733–2734. https://doi.org/10.1016/j.ajem.2020.04.025

Xu, T., Pujara, S., Sutton, S., & Rhee, M. (2018). Telemedicine in the management of type 1 diabetes. *Preventing Chronic Disease*, *15*. https://doi.org/10.5888/pcd15.170168

Zhou, X., Snoswell, C. L., Harding, L. E., et al. (2020). The role of telehealth in reducing the mental health burden from COVID-19. *Telemedicine Journal and E-Health*, *26*(4), 377–379. https://doi.org/10.1089/tmj.2020.0068

SECTION 2

Telehealth

4

Foundations of Telehealth: Lessons from Telehealth Practice in the United States

Karen S. Rheuban, MD

"Advances in the delivery of a broad range of virtual care models, propelled by the COVID-19 public health emergency, have led to a paradigm shift in telehealth-supported care transformations."

OBJECTIVES

1. Understand telehealth definitions.
2. Understand foundational principles of telehealth practice.
3. Review different models of care.
4. Describe relevant legal and privacy regulations for telehealth (AAMC Domain VI, 2021).

CHAPTER OUTLINE

INTRODUCTION TO TELEHEALTH

Digital-age healthcare technologies offer tools and support processes that improve access and quality via transformational care delivery mechanisms. Demand for innovative solutions has been driven by an aging population, high rates of chronic illness, geographic and socio-demographic disparities in access to care, increasing numbers of patients seeking care in the face of health professional workforce shortages, and most recently, a devastating global pandemic. Not specialties in and of themselves, telemedicine and telehealth offer tools to address the significant challenges of access, quality, and cost—the "triple aim" articulated by the Institute for Healthcare Improvement (Institute for Healthcare Improvement, n.d.).

Telehealth means a mode of delivering healthcare services through the use of telecommunications technologies, including but not limited to asynchronous and synchronous technology, and remote patient monitoring technology, by a healthcare practitioner to a patient or a practitioner at a different physical location than the healthcare practitioner (ATA, 2020).

Telehealth generally refers to a broad range of health-related services across a wide range of disciplines supported by telecommunications technology that includes telemedicine, as well as health-related distance learning, remote patient monitoring, call centers, consumer-facing virtual and e-health applications, and other services that enhance health but do not necessarily represent the delivery of clinical care.

There are a number of definitions of telemedicine and telehealth used by federal and state agencies. The US Health Resource and Services Administration, home to the federal Office for the Advancement of Telehealth defines telehealth as: "the use of electronic information and telecommunication technologies to support long-distance clinical healthcare, patient and professional health-related education, health administration, and public health." https://www.hrsa.gov/rural-health/telehealth/what-is-telehealth.

State definitions vary, and often include definitions in code such as that of Virginia. Telemedicine services as it pertains to the delivery of health care services, means the use of electronic technology or media, including interactive audio or video, for the purpose of diagnosing or treating a patient, providing remote patient monitoring services, or consulting with other health care providers regarding a patient's diagnosis or treatment, regardless of the originating site and whether the patient is accompanied by a health care provider at the time such services are provided. Telemedicine services does not include an audio-only telephone, electronic mail message, facsimile transmission, or online questionnaire. Nothing in this section shall preclude coverage for a service that is not a telemedicine service, including services delivered through real-time audio-only telephone. (State of Virginia, 24 March, 2021).

Accordingly, the reader is advised to ensure programmatic efforts align with both federal and state definitions, laws, and regulations. Additional relevant terminologies relate to the location of the patient (referred to as the "originating site") and the location of the provider (referred to as the "distant site"). Patient originating sites may include healthcare facilities, the home, the workplace, schools, or other locations. Distant-site provider locations could include healthcare facilities, offices, or even the home of the provider (http://thesource.american-telemed.org/resources/telemedicine-glossary).

Modalities of telemedicine services include synchronous services delivered in real time, asynchronous services through which medical images or data are transferred for interpretation and clinical decision-making, or blended models that incorporate both.

The services and modalities used include:

- live interactive services that connect a "remote" patient, caregiver, or provider in real time with a distant-site provider using audiovisual telecommunications technology functioning in lieu of an in-person encounter;
- store-and-forward technologies which enable the asynchronous transmission of medical information, images, and other data through secure electronic formats to support a clinical diagnosis and patient management;
- remote patient monitoring (RPM) tools and services that utilize digital technologies to collect physiologic data from patients in one location (generally the home) which are subsequently transmitted electronically and securely to healthcare providers;
- remote communications technology-based services, which are services not defined as telemedicine within Medicare (because they do not have an in-person equivalent) and include provider-to-provider asynchronous communications (eConsults), brief check-ins with established patients, chronic care management, remote physiologic monitoring services, and e-visits connecting patients with their providers through an electronic portal; and
- m-Health, which represents the delivery of any of the above services through a mobile platform.

TELEHEALTH MODELS OF CARE

Models of telehealth-supported care are as diverse as healthcare in general (Darkins et al., 2008; Kvedar et al., 2014; Lustig, 2012).

These include connecting tertiary and quaternary healthcare facilities (academic or otherwise) to other facilities in a hub-and-spoke model to provide specialty care services. Other models include "networks of networks," as has been developed in the province-wide Ontario Telehealth Network, driven in some cases by governmental or quasi-governmental entities leveraging regional or statewide investments in broadband communications services and health information exchanges. Consortium models have been developed that include contracting to enhance collaboration between academic providers and other entities, both within and beyond state borders (e.g., prison telemedicine). Payer- and employer-driven models have been developed in the urgent care/primary care direct-to-consumer market. Private telemedicine specialty care companies offer contracted services across multiple states to provide services such as tele-stroke, telepsychiatry, critical care, or remote monitoring.

Clinical consultations and follow-up visits have long represented the traditional model of telemedicine. Nearly all healthcare specialties have applicability and have contributed to the evidence base for telehealth, across the continuum from prenatal care to end-of-life care, including acute care and chronic disease management. Specialties such as critical care, primary care, emergency services, surgery, pediatrics and pediatric subspecialties, psychiatry, radiology, neurology and neurosurgery, dermatology, ophthalmology, cardiology, obstetrics, pulmonary medicine, gastroenterology, infectious diseases, orthopedics, endocrinology, plastic surgery, pathology, genetics, and rehabilitation have made significant contributions to the evidence base for telemedicine. Other nonphysician disciplines and professions are

Telemedicine Can Facilitate a Broad Range of Interactions, Using Different Devices and Modalities

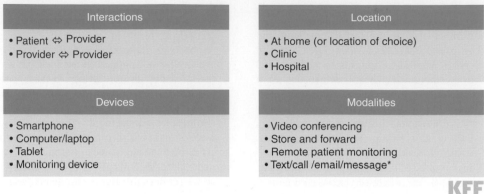

Interactions	Location
• Patient ⇔ Provider • Provider ⇔ Provider	• At home (or location of choice) • Clinic • Hospital

Devices	Modalities
• Smartphone • Computer/laptop • Tablet • Monitoring device	• Video conferencing • Store and forward • Remote patient monitoring • Text/call /email/message*

Notes: *Text/call/email/messaging are not considered telemedicine by many definitions.

Fig. 4.1 Telehealth modalities, interactions and devices. (Source: https://www.kff.org/womens-health-policy/issue-brief/telemedicine-in-sexual-and-reproductive-health/)

Telehealth continuum

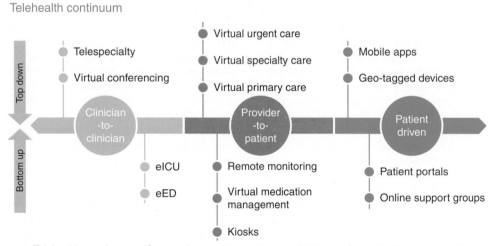

Fig. 4.2 Telehealth continuum. (Source: https://blog.webex.com/video-conferencing/improving-patient-care-and-coordination-with-video-conferencing-and-team-collaboration-tools/)

fully engaged in telehealth, including but not limited to nursing, dentistry, pharmacy, behavioral health, social work, nutrition services, physical and occupational therapy, speech and language services, genetic counseling, and home health. These care models can be accomplished using either synchronous or asynchronous telemedicine technologies, the outcomes of which have been well documented in the peer-reviewed literature (Bashshur et al., 2014; Dimmick et al., 2000; Grabowski & O'Malley, 2014). Extensive evidence published in the peer-reviewed literature demonstrates that telemedicine improves clinical outcomes and lowers the cost of care, although overprescribing of antibiotics in direct-to-consumer models has been demonstrated (Agency for Healthcare Research and Quality, 2016; Uscher-Pines et al., 2015; Uscher-Pines et al., 2016).

Elements that contribute to the successful adoption of any telemedicine program include the establishment of consistent workflows, training of practitioners and staff, technology acquisition, broadband connectivity, tracking of clinical and process quality metrics, workforce capacity, and careful analyses of outcomes, including return on investment. These must be considered in the context of organizational mission and programmatic alignment with that mission. Practice guidelines have been developed by many advocacy organizations (AAFP, n.d.; AAP, 2017; AMA, 2015, 2016; Daniel & Sulmasy, 2015; Gough et al., 2015).

International Care Delivery Models

Telehealth solutions have been broadly deployed both for international systems of care and in global philanthropic models. The reader is advised to be aware of relevant statutes and regulations governing telehealth practice, to include scope of practice, licensure, reimbursement, telecommunications service availability, and privacy and security laws (Alverson, 2018).

One of the longest serving charities focused on improving access to care via telemedicine is the Swinfen Charitable Trust, based in the United Kingdom. Since 1998, this organization has utilized a large international network of vetted volunteer (primarily academic medical) consultants to support store-and-forward consultation requests from providers in underserved countries. Other charitable organizations utilizing telemedicine include Médecins Sans Frontières, Shriners, AMD Global Medicine, Project Hope, Medical Mission for Children, Project ECHO (Extension for Community Healthcare Outcomes), and Partners in Health, to name just a few.

WORKFORCE IMPLICATIONS

In the United States the Association of American Medical Colleges has projected a physician shortage ranging between 61,700 and 94,700 physicians by the year 2025, with particular shortages in primary care (Rheuban & Shipman, 2018). In addition, the aging of our population with increased rates of chronic illness places a particular strain on the existing physician workforce and need for primary care providers. The urban predilection for specialty providers also results in barriers in access to specialty care for rural patients (AAMC, 2016; Hooker & Muchow, 2014; HRSA, 2015; Rheuban & Shipman, 2018; US Department of Health and Human Services, 2014, 2016).

There has been incremental significant growth in the numbers of advanced practice providers, including physician assistants and advanced practice nurses (Hooker & Muchow, 2014; US Department of Health and Human Services, 2014). It is estimated that by 2025 the supply of physician assistants will increase by more than 50% (Rheuban & Shipman, 2018). Similarly, the number of advanced practice nurses has more than doubled over the last 10 years, as has the overall nursing workforce. Increased demand for behavioral health providers, including psychologists, counselors, and social workers, has resulted in new models of care delivery, including behavioral health being integrated into primary care. Pharmacists have taken on expanded roles in medication management and patient education. A broad range of allied health professionals, such as physical therapists, occupational therapists, and dieticians, are now part of care teams along with community health workers, care coordinators, medical assistants, scribes, and health coaches.

Each of the aforementioned providers may offer virtual care within their scope of practice. Advanced practice providers may practice independently, depending on state law, or through collaborating agreements with physicians. Practice through virtual modalities must align with in-person practice regulations. Technology innovations have enabled multiple parties to participate in virtual visits simultaneously or through virtual handoffs in care, supporting team-based care delivery models. Similarly, remote supervision models enable trainee and mentor-supported virtual visits. Community health workers and home health providers also utilize telehealth technologies to support patients at home in team-based models of care. As the healthcare delivery system evolves, it is critical to ensure that all providers within the healthcare ecosystem adapt to new models of care and are trained accordingly to incorporate virtual solutions in a coordinated fashion.

TECHNOLOGY CONSIDERATIONS

Telecommunications Technologies

Telecommunications technologies provide the requisite communications infrastructure over which telehealth solutions are driven so as to enable connected care (Rheuban & Shipman, 2018). Video-based services, store-and-forward services, and mobile technologies all require sufficient bandwidth to transfer images and data in a timely fashion. Broadband networks provide the foundation for telehealth solutions and can be wired or wireless, fixed or mobile, satellite or terrestrial. Network availability and performance is more challenging for mobile services than for fixed broadband and this relates in part to spectrum availability. Transitioning from 3G to 5G networks provides improved broadband performance. Greater demand and innovation have led to both federal and private investments in broadband services, including low-orbit satellite technologies and 5G networks.

Videoconferencing

In simple terms, a synchronous videoconference is a meeting that connects two parties at a distance and allows the participants to see and hear one another in real time. This can be accomplished with a camera, microphone, and speakers, and either a software program that encodes and decodes the stream (codec) or via a software program (a "bridge") that manages the exchange between participants. "Point-to-point" videoconferencing connects one party with another, whereas "multipoint" video calls require central software/hardware programs that can control and manage participants joining with different communications protocols and connection speeds, converting those protocols to a common language and ensuring a functional connection. Communications protocols may include H.323 (ISDN), H.264 (IP), and SIP (Session Initiation Protocol), in addition to other proprietary audio-video compression protocols. WebRTC—a real-time communications service layered on top of an open standard through which voice, video, and data services are implemented— has been increasingly incorporated into telemedicine solutions.

Bandwidth

Bandwidth is the rate of data transfer measured in bits per second (bps) and ranges from low bandwidth of kilobits per second (Kbps) to high-bandwidth service in the ranges of millions or billions of bits per second (megabits or gigabits per second; Mbps or Gbps). Different telemedicine applications require different bandwidths; for example, text messaging at <1000 bps, a phone call at 5600 bps (56 kbps), standard-definition video at 1 Mbps, or high-definition video at 4 Mbps. Within a network, the ultimate bandwidth for the video connection is limited to the lowest bandwidth of the end-user. Other factors impacting performance include the level and type of compression used, packet loss, latency, and jitter. The National Broadband Plan commissioned by the Federal Communications Commission (FCC) established aspirational goals for bandwidth allocated for a wide range of healthcare connections. The Commission articulated the progress toward that goal in 2016 (FCC, 2011, 2016).

Mobile Medical Applications

Mobile medical applications are software applications and devices that leverage the portability offered by mobile technologies. Some target health and wellness, some capture and incorporate biometric data, and others facilitate the delivery of care to patients. The FDA has formally defined a mobile platform as "commercial off-the-shelf computing platforms, with or without wireless connectivity that are handheld in nature" (US Food and Drug Administration, 2015) and a mobile application as a "software application that can be executed (run) on a mobile platform (i.e., a handheld commercial off-the-shelf computing platform, with or without wireless connectivity), or a web-based software application that is tailored to a mobile platform but is executed on a server". It has provided guidance that a mobile medical app is a mobile app that meets the definition of device in section 201(h) of the Federal Food, Drug and Cosmetic Act and either is intended to be used as an accessory to a regulated medical device or to transform a mobile platform into a regulated medical device. The FDA considers the intended use of the mobile app in order to determine whether it meets the definition of a "device." If an app is intended for use in performing a function for

diagnosis or treatment, it is considered a device regardless of the platform on which it runs. There are more non-FDA-approved apps than approved ones, and many are freely downloadable for consumer use. Users (providers and patients) need to be cautious with these apps, however, as they are not often validated or tested for reliability.

Electronic Medical Record Integration/Health Information Exchange

The exchange of patient medical information provided via telemedicine is optimized when integrated into a patient's medical record, and information is most easily exchanged between providers when documentation conforms to other standards for electronic records, such as Health Level 7 (HL7) or Fast Healthcare Interoperability Resources (FHIR), an application programming interface (API) for exchanging electronic health records. Some telehealth providers have utilized electronic medical record (EMR) vendors that have integrated telehealth solutions into their platform (including video services, scheduling, documentation, and billing) that can be exchanged between providers both within and external to the provider's system; and others have utilized cloud-based solutions to effect and document the telemedicine encounter. Standards and guidelines developed by the ATA and many of the specialty advocacy organizations call for documentation of the encounter within a medical record and, where appropriate and with the patient's consent, sharing of the information with the patient's referring provider/medical home.

Peripheral Devices

Telemedicine devices and applications that support patient encounters beyond a video-based service alone to allow the clinician to comport to the standard of in-person care include electronic stethoscopes, otoscopes, ophthalmoscopes, dermatoscopes, colposcopes, spirometers, electronic scales, glucometers, sphygmomanometers, electrocardiograms, thermometers, and a range of other digitally configured integrated examination tools. Some devices require the presence of a clinician or a tele-presenter, while others can be utilized by patients. Interoperability of devices plays an important role. The *Continua Health Alliance* is an industry collaborative advocacy organization designed to advance and support standards of interoperability of devices, sensors, and other connected health tools (Continua Health Alliance, n.d.). The federally funded National Telehealth Technology Assessment Resource Center (TTAC) offers an independent assessment of telehealth technologies and guidance for providers and systems seeking information related to technology appropriate to the setting desired (TTAC, n.d.). FDA guidance indicates that when performing a function for diagnosis or treatment, any device, regardless of the platform on which it runs, is regulated as a medical device, and as such is subject to regulation. "The FDA also encourages mobile medical app manufacturers to search FDA's public databases, such as the 'Product Classification' database and the '510(k) Premarket Notification' database, to determine the level of regulation for a given device and for the most up-to-date information about the relevant regulatory requirements."

Telemedicine improves patient triage, reduces the burden of travel for care, fosters more timely access to care, and provides tools that support patient engagement and self-management via a growing variety of applications and services. These may be supported through the use of two-way videoconferencing either with or without the use of peripheral remote examination devices, store-and-forward asynchronous technologies, remote monitoring tools, and hybrids representing each of these models.

Advancements in state and federal public policy, coupled with greater engagement by providers, payers, employers, and consumers, have led to new paradigms of care enhanced by telemedicine. Federal and state actions and waivers implemented during the COVID-19 public health emergency, and by necessity, have resulted in a dramatic increase in telehealth services.

IMPACT OF THE COVID-19 PUBLIC HEALTH EMERGENCY

The COVID-19 pandemic has resulted in a massive scaling up of the use of telehealth worldwide by clinicians in small practices and large healthcare systems as an essential tool to maintain access to care while reducing exposure of patients and providers alike. Telehealth solutions have been adopted to maintain ambulatory visits, to screen patients for COVID-19, to monitor patients with COVID-19 through RPM tools, to conserve personal protective equipment in isolation settings, to reduce the need for emergency room visits through virtual urgent care models, and to enhance access to specialty care services, including in congregate care settings such as long-term care. Through federal and state actions (waivers, executive orders), many of the pre-COVID-19 barriers to adoption of telehealth in Medicare, Medicaid, and commercial insurance plans have been eliminated during the public health emergency. Enabled by these and other recent regulatory and statutory changes, and by necessity, patients and providers have turned to digital health platforms, devices, and services to provide and receive care in place to avoid unnecessary exposure to the novel coronavirus.

Prepandemic policy barriers in the United States include coverage and payment restrictions, particularly in fee-for-service models, licensure, broadband availability, and federal and state prescribing regulations. Limited training and lack of investment in telehealth platforms by providers and healthcare systems presented additional barriers to the scaling of telehealth (Centers for Medicare and Medicaid Services, 2018). Patient satisfaction data, as reported by Press Ganey and Associates, have demonstrated exceptionally high rates of patient satisfaction with telehealth during the COVID-19 pandemic (Press Ganey, 2020).

These recent telehealth flexibilities in Medicare tied to the public health emergency, along with state actions in Medicaid, by gubernatorial executive orders, and additional actions by commercial insurers, all have played a critical role in helping to maintain access to primary and specialty healthcare services. This exponentially scaled coverage expansion during the COVID-19 public health emergency will further enable Health and Human Services (HHS) to study the cost-effectiveness, clinical outcomes, and any incidents of fraud or abuse related to telemedicine services covered by federal payment programs.

UNITED STATES PUBLIC POLICIES

Medicare, Medicaid, and Private Payer Coverage of Telehealth

Prior to the COVID-19 public health emergency, Medicare reimbursement of telehealth services provided to fee-for-service beneficiaries remained limited due to the 1834(m) restrictions of the Social Security Act. The 21st Century Cures Act directed the Centers for Medicare and Medicaid Services (CMS) to provide an update on telehealth services provided to Medicare beneficiaries. Claims data analyses demonstrated that between 2014 and 2016, only 0.25% of the more than 35 million Medicare beneficiaries in the fee-for-service program utilized a telehealth service (CMS, 2018). That report suggested that the most significant statutory restrictions to the utilization of telehealth included: (1) the requirement that the patient's originating site be rural and (2) that the home is not an eligible originating site. With the changes to policy and regulation during the pandemic, the Office of the Assistant Secretary for Planning and Evaluation (ASPE) reported that utilization of telemedicine for primary care visits jumped from 0.1% of visits in February 2020 to 44% of visits in May 2020 (ASPE, 2020).

During the public health emergency of the COVID-19 pandemic, provisions of the CONNECT for Health Act were included in the Coronavirus Preparedness and Response Supplemental Appropriations Act and the Coronavirus Aid Relief and Economic Security Act, giving the Secretary of Health and Human Services authority to waive telehealth requirements under Section 1834(m) of the Social Security Act, and allowing Federally Qualified Health Centers (FQHCs) and Rural Health Clinics (RHCs) to provide distant site telehealth services. CMS issued regulatory waivers and Interim Final Rules in March and April 2020 related to the provision of Medicare telehealth services. Importantly, these COVID-19 public health emergency waivers eliminated geographic restrictions, allowed the home as an eligible originating site, expanded eligible distant site providers, enabled FQHCs and RHCs to serve as both eligible originating and distant sites, expanded covered CPT (Current Procedural Terminology) codes, and allowed hospitals to charge a (limited) facility fee, along with other important changes.

Importantly, the activation of telephone codes enabled greater continuity of care, particularly for patients for whom lack of access to broadband or satisfactory video remains a barrier. The adoption of alternative payment models in the public and private sector offers an alternative to telehealth coverage restrictions.

Fifty state Medicaid programs plus the District of Columbia provide some form of reimbursement for the delivery of telehealth-facilitated care to Medicaid beneficiaries. Medicaid innovations adopted by many states in addition to video-based telemedicine consults and follow-up visits include coverage for remote monitoring, home telehealth, and store-and-forward services. Most states have mirrored the Medicare flexibilities in Medicaid to enable continuity of care for children, pregnant women, and medically complex patients.

Forty-two states plus the District of Columbia require private insurers to cover telehealth services, although not all at parity with in-person services. Many US employer-based health plans in the United States (Employee Retirement Income Security Act plans, not bound by state reimbursement policies) have chosen to cover telehealth services for their covered employees. Post-public health emergency, most commercial plans expanded coverage for telehealth services aligned with Medicare, with variable sunset dates either for elimination of coverage tied to the public health emergency or eliminated waivers of co-pays at variable dates.

Licensure

States have the authority to regulate the practice of medicine within their boundaries. Most require out-of-state clinicians providing telehealth services to be licensed in the state where the patient resides. The Federation of State Medical Boards (FSMB) offers a process that allows state medical boards to retain their disciplinary authority, while expediting the licensing process for physicians seeking to practice in multiple states. Some states offer other models of expedited licensure or reciprocity. During the COVID-19 public health emergency, through the waiver process, Medicare allowed for reimbursement for services provided to patients in states where the practitioner was not licensed, so long as that individual practitioner held a valid license in another state and was enrolled in the Medicare program. By executive order, many states have implemented similar waivers of licensure during the COVID-19 public health emergency.

Health Insurance Portability and Accountability Act Privacy and Security

During the public health emergency, the Office of Civil Rights (OCR) issued a waiver of enforcement discretion against healthcare providers who in good faith utilized non-Health Insurance Portability and Accountability Act (HIPAA)-compliant applications to connect with their patients. States may have additional HIPAA privacy and security laws, and as such the federal waiver does not eliminate risk for providers, who may still be subject to state enforcement action.

Prescribing Regulations

The Drug Enforcement Administration (DEA) regulates prescribing of controlled substances as it relates to the establishment of a doctor-patient relationship resulting in prescribing. Many states defer to federal law; the DEA, by law, is currently tasked with developing a special telemedicine registration process.

Broadband Access

The FCC, as a provision of the Telecommunications Act of 1996, established the Rural Health Care Program under the Universal Services Administrative Corporation (USAC). This program has provided support for critical broadband infrastructure to healthcare facilities. The FCC and many of the states themselves track broadband availability, including to the census tract level. The FCC Connect2Health Task Force mapped broadband availability and health status indicators, and suggested that lack of broadband is indeed a health equity issue. The FCC reports that 53% of rural Americans (22 million people) lack access to sufficient broadband to support benchmarked service as articulated in the National Broadband Plan. The Commission recently voted to establish two additional programs—the $200 million COVID-19 Telehealth Program, funded by the Coronavirus Aid, Relief, and Economic Security (CARES) Act, and the $100 million Connected Care Pilot Program— designed to enable healthcare providers and systems to deploy broadband to the homes of their patients. Other federal and state programs have supported broadband expansion, particularly in rural and underserved areas.

CONCLUSION

Telehealth is an essential tool to address the significant challenges of providing access to high-quality care regardless of patient location. Telehealth tools and models of care delivery have been demonstrated to favorably impact both acute and chronic illness, reduce disparities, mitigate workforce shortages, improve population health, and lower the cost of care.

The COVID-19 pandemic has demonstrated that telehealth plays a critical role in ensuring access to care, reducing patient and provider exposure, protecting vulnerable populations, conserving personal protective equipment, and improving clinical outcomes with high rates of patient satisfaction. Broader adoption of telehealth will require expansion of workforce training, education of patients, expansion of broadband communications services, and continued analyses of costs and outcomes that enable further integration of telehealth into everyday care.

In the digital era, it is imperative to advance evidence-based care delivery models and promulgate policies that foster high-quality, sustainable telehealth solutions that empower patients, providers, and payers to adopt 21st-century models of care.

KEY POINTS

Models of telehealth-supported care are as diverse as healthcare in general.

- The COVID-19 pandemic has resulted in a massive scaling of the use of telehealth worldwide as an essential tool to maintain access to care while reducing exposure of patients and providers alike.
- Broader adoption of telehealth will require expansion of training of the workforce, education of patients, expansion of broadband communications services, and continued analyses of costs and outcomes that enable further integration of telehealth into everyday care

Relevant guidelines:

- American Telemedicine Association. (2015). ATA practice guidelines for live, on-demand primary and urgent care.
- American Medical Association. (2014). Report of the Council on Medical Service: coverage of and payment for telemedicine.
- American Medical Association. (2016). Report of the Council on Judicial and Ethical Affairs, Guidance for Ethical Practice in Telemedicine
- American College of Physicians. (2015). Policy recommendations to guide the use of telemedicine in primary care settings: American College of Physicians position paper. https://www.acpjournals.org/doi/10.7326/m15-0498
- American Academy of Family Physicians. (2015). https://www.graham-center.org/content/dam/rgc/documents/publications-reports/reports/RGC2015Telehealth Report.pdf
- American Academy of Pediatrics. (2017). Operating procedures for pediatric telehealth. *Pediatrics*, *140*(2).
- American Telemedicine Association. (2021). Practice guidelines http://hub.americantelemed.org/resources/telemedicine-practice-guidelines

REFERENCES

AAMC. (2021). *Telehealth competencies across the learning continuum. AAMC New and Emerging Areas in Medicine Series.* Washington, DC: AAMC.

AAMC Workforce Statement. (2016). https://www.aamc.org/media/54681/download.

Agency for Healthcare Research and Quality. (2016). *Effective health care program.* Rockville, MD. https://accessmedicine.mhmedical.com/content.aspx?bookid=2217&sectionid=187795630.

Alverson, D. C. (2018). The role of telehealth in international humanitarian outreach. In K. Rheuban, K. E. A. Rheuban, & E. A. Krupinski (Eds.), *Understanding telehealth.* McGraw-Hill. https://accessmedicine.mhmedical.com/content.aspx?bookid=2217&sectionid=187795630.

American Academy of Family Physicians. (2015). Klink, K., Coffman, M., Moore M., et al. https://www.graham-center.org/content/dam/rgc/documents/publications-reports/reports/RGC2015Telehealth Report.pdf.

American Academy of Pediatrics. (2017). McSwain, D., Bernard, J., et al., Operating Procedures for Pediatric Telehealth. *Telemed J E Health.* 23(9):699–706.

American Medical Association. (2014). Report of the Council on medical service: Coverage of and payment for telemedicine. *CMS Report*, *7*, A-14. https://www.ama-assn.org/practice-management/digital/new-telemedicine-policy-lays-out-principles-coverage-payment.

American Medical Association. (2016). *Report of the Council on Judicial and Ethical Affairs, guidance for ethical practice in telemedicine.* https://www.ama-assn.org/practice-management/digital/telemedicine-prompts-new-ethical-ground-rules-physicians.

American Telemedicine Association. (2020). https://www.americantelemed.org/wp-content/uploads/2020/10/ATA-_Medical-Practice-10-5-20.pdf.

ASPE. (2020). *Medicare beneficiary use of telehealth visits: Early data from the start of the COVID-19 pandemic.* https://aspe.hhs.gov/pdf-report/medicare-beneficiary-use-telehealth. [Accessed 31 October 2021].

Bashshur, R. L., Shannon, G. W., Smith, B. R., et al. (2014). The empirical foundations of telemedicine interventions for chronic disease management. *Telemedicine Journal and e-Health, 20*(9), 769–800. https://doi.org/10.1089/tmj.2014.9981.

Centers for Medicare and Medicaid Services. (2018). *Information on Medicare telehealth*. https://www.cms.gov/About-CMS/Agency-Information/OMH/Downloads/Information-on-Medicare-Telehealth-Report.pdf. [Accessed 31 October 2021].

Continua health alliance (n.d.). http://www.pchalliance.org/continua.

Daniel, H., & Sulmasy, L. S. (2015). Policy recommendations to guide the use of telemedicine in primary care settings: An American College of physicians position paper. *Annals of Internal Medicine, 163*(10), 787–789. https://www.acpjournals.org/doi/10.7326/M15-0498.

Darkins, A., Ryan, P., Kobb, R., et al. (2008). Care coordination/home telehealth: The systematic implementation of health informatics, home telehealth, and disease management to support the care of veteran patients with chronic conditions. *Telemedicine Journal and e-Health, 14*(10), 1118–1126. https://doi.org/10.1089/tmj.2008.0021.

Dimmick, S. L., Mustaleski, C., Burgiss, S. G., et al. (2000). A case study of benefits & potential savings in rural home telemedicine. *Home Healthcare Nurse, 18*(2), 124–135. https://doi.org/10.1097/00004045-200002000-00013.

Federal Communications Commission. (2011). *The National broadband plan: Connecting America. Chapter 10: Healthcare.* Washington, DC: Federal Communications Commission. https://www.fcc.gov/general/national-broadband-plan.

Federal Communications Commission. (2016). *2016 Broadband progress report.* Washington, DC: Federal Communications Commission. https://www.fcc.gov/reports-research/reports/broadband-progress-reports/2016-broadband-progress-report. [Accessed 31 October 2021].

Ganey, Press (2020). *Press Ganey Releases Landmark Telemedicine Report, Revealing New Consumer Insights for Providers to Meet Patients' Evolving Needs.* http://about.pressganey.com/about/press-releases/press-release-details/2020/Press-Ganey-Releases-Landmark-Telemedicine-Report-Revealing-New-Consumer-Insights-for-Providers-to-Meet-Patients-Evolving-Needs/default.aspx.

Gough, F., Budhrani, S., Cohn, E., et al. (2015). ATA practice guidelines for live, on-demand primary and urgent care. *Telemedicine Journal and e-Health, 21*(3), 233–241. https://doi.org/10.1089/tmj.2015.0008.

Grabowski, D. C., & O'Malley, A. J. (2014). Use of telemedicine can reduce hospitalizations of nursing home residents and generate savings for medicare. *Health Affairs, 33*(2), 244–250. https://doi.org/10.1377/hlthaff.2013.0922.

Health Resources and Services Administration/National Center for Health Workforce Analysis; Substance Abuse and Mental Health Services Administration/Office of Policy, Planning, and Innovation. (2015). *National projections of supply and demand for behavioral health practitioners: 2013–2025.* Rockville, MD. https://bhw.hrsa.gov/data-research/projecting-health-workforce-supply-demand/behavioral-health.

Hooker, R. S., & Muchow, A. N. (2014). Supply of physician assistants: 2013-2026. *Journal of the American Academy of PAs, 27*(3), 39–45. https://doi.org/10.1097/01.JAA.0000443969.69352.4a.

Institute for healthcare Improvement. (n.d.). the IHI triple aim. http://www.ihi.org/engage/initiatives/tripleaim/pages/default.aspx. [Accessed 31 October 2021].

Kvedar, J., Coye, M. J., & Everett, W. (2014). Connected health: A review of technologies and strategies to improve patient care with telemedicine and telehealth. *Health Affairs, 33*(2), 194–199. https://doi.org/10.1377/hlthaff.2013.0992.

Lustig, T. A. (2012). *The role of telehealth in an evolving health care environment: Workshop summary.* National Academies Press.

Rheuban, K., & Shipman, S. (2018). Workforce, definitions, and models. In K. Rheuban, K. E. A. Rheuban, & E. A. Krupinski (Eds.), *Understanding telehealth.* McGraw-Hill. https://accessmedicine.mhmedical.com/content.aspx?bookid=2217&sectionid=187794500.

State of Virginia. (Virginia State Law § 38.2-3418.16.) Coverage for telemedicine services. http://law.lis.virginia.gov/vacode/title38.2/chapter34/section38.2-3418.16/. [Accessed 24 March 2021].

TTAC (n.d.). The National Telehealth Technology Assessment Resource Center. https://telehealthtechnology.org/. [Accessed 31 October 2021].

Uscher-Pines, L., Mulcahy, A., Cowling, D., et al. (2015). Antibiotic prescribing for acute respiratory infections in direct-to-consumer telemedicine visits. *JAMA Internal Medicine, 175*(7), 1234–1235. https://doi.org/10.1001/jamainternmed.2015.2024.

Uscher-Pines, L., Mulcahy, A., Cowling, D., et al. (2016). Access and quality of care in direct-to-consumer telemedicine. *Telemedicine Journal and e-Health, 22*(4), 282–287. https://doi.org/10.1089/tmj.2015.0079.

US Department of Health and Human Services, Health Resources and Services Administration, National Center for Health Workforce Analysis. (2016). *National and regional projections of supply and demand for primary care practitioners,* 2013–2025. https://bhw.hrsa.gov/sites/default/files/bureau-health-workforce/data-research/primary-care-national-projections-2013-2025.pdf.

US Department of Health and Human Services, Health Resources and Services Administration, National Center for Health Workforce Analysis. (2014a). In *Highlights from the 2012 National Sample Survey of Nurse Practitioners.* Rockville, MD: US Department of Health and Human Services. https://bhw.hrsa.gov/data-research/access-data-tools/national-sample-survey-registered-nurse-practitioners.

US Department of Health and Human Services Health Resources and Services Administration National Center for Health Workforce Analysis. (2014b). *The future of the nursing workforce: National- and state-level projections, 2012–2025.* Rockville, MD.

US Department of Health and Human Services. US Food & Drug Administration. (2015). *Medical devices.* Silver Spring, MD. https://www.fda.gov/medical-devices/digital-health-center-excellence/device-software-functions-including-mobile-medical-applications.

Establishing Telehealth Programs in Clinical Practice

Edward Marx, BS, MS

"You have to be careful if you do not know where you are going because you might not get there."

Yogi Berra

OBJECTIVES

1. Identify critical factors essential in the development, implementation, management, and evaluation of telehealth programs to achieve sustainability, using the strengths of Interprofessional Communication (IPEC CC1-8)
2. Describe how human-centered design and user experience factor into customer satisfaction to include patients, families, and clinicians.
3. Learn the fundamentals and necessity of business plans to ensure adequate funding and investment to include telehealth revenue models and drivers.
4. Determine best practices for operational models to include the leverage of agile methodologies to ensure efficient and effective operations.
5. Harness the disciplines of measurement and transparency to ensure an understanding of baseline clinical, operational, and financial environments.

CHAPTER OUTLINE

KEY TERMS

Digital transformation is a foundational change in how an organization delivers value to its customers leveraging modern technical capabilities

Telehealth refers broadly to electronic and telecommunications technologies and services used to provide care and services at-a-distance.

61

Telemedicine is the practice of medicine using technology to deliver care at a distance. A physician in one location uses a telecommunications infrastructure to deliver care to a patient at a distant site. Telehealth is different from telemedicine in that it refers to a broader scope of remote health care services than telemedicine. Telemedicine refers specifically to remote clinical services, while telehealth can refer to remote non-clinical services.

Video conferencing is a type of online meeting where two or more people engage in a live audio and visual call.

INTRODUCTION

The purpose of this chapter is to cover key factors and techniques that are significant for establishing telehealth programs in clinical practice. Given the relative immaturity of this space, there is no previously accepted best practice. That said, the chapter takes advantage of precedent and experience while covering foundational elements required to enable a thriving telehealth practice based on interprofessional teamwork. While there is acceptable variation in approach, the model that follows helps decrease risks while increasing the odds of success. The foundation is built on interprofessional teamwork, culture and change management, technology deployment, training, agile operations, legal and regulatory considerations, business planning, marketing, and finally, performance monitoring. Clinical care in the postpandemic era must be efficient, effective, and focused on human-centered design. Successful telehealth practice merges the best of quality care and technology while ensuring the most engaged experience possible for patients, their families, and clinicians.

CASE STUDY: WIMBLEDON CLINICS, ENGLAND

While most available evidence suggests that the volume of telehealth visits will fall substantially over the next year or so, as the COVID-19 pandemic loses its grip on the world, in some cases delivering telehealth services during lockdown has fostered acceptance of virtual care among providers as a long-term strategy (Zieger, 2020). This case study describes how one UK-based practice created a model for implementing virtual visits and began preparing for a telehealth-driven future.

When COVID-19 hit, leaders at sports medicine–focused Wimbledon Clinics decided to get into telemedicine as quickly as possible. Once they made the decision, the group transitioned to virtual care in one week. The practice's leaders were motivated by insurers willing to pay for telehealth services during the pandemic lockdown.

The first thing the clinic's telehealth team did was to get a comprehensive look at existing administrative processes for handling in-person visits. The group spent 5 days writing down those processes and determining how to perform these services virtually (Zieger, 2020). Their efforts touched every department and required physicians to adopt new approaches to care management. They created a package of information for clinicians on how to handle a video call, record notes, get into online records, and share scanned information.

Clinic managers also examined what patients might want from telemedicine visits. This involved equipping clinicians to ask questions that would help patients share their ideal telehealth experience (Zieger, 2020). Managers also built a team of practice owners focused on improving telehealth delivery and planning for future efforts. They took care to choose the right video platform for conducting video visits; project leads checked Skype, Zoom, and Webex, ultimately deciding that Zoom worked best for their purposes.

When the clinic surveyed members about their telemedicine experiences, it received positive responses: 95% of respondents reported that the video consult was worthwhile or very worthwhile, and 60% said they would value virtual care options at any time, not just during the lockdown (Zieger, 2020). The managers decided to offer video consults as a permanent service.

Many elderly patients said they weren't comfortable with telehealth and were unclear on the value for them. This experience needs to be evaluated further and design improvements made to better accommodate the elderly. Regardless, the efforts Wimbledon Clinics made to map their offline processes to telehealth are commendable. When leaders take a holistic approach to include care redesign, telehealth will be increasingly successful.

CASE STUDY: ALTAMED, UNITED STATES

Nonprofit healthcare company AltaMed Health Services was founded as the East Los Angeles Barrio Free Clinic in 1969, with a mission to provide healthcare to the underserved Latino and multiethnic population of east Los Angeles. There was a lack of healthcare available in this area but today AltaMed is one of the largest community health centers in the country, serving nearly 300,000 patients with more than 1,000,000 visits a year (Kianickova, 2020). AltaMed serves everyone and anyone, independent of their ability to pay or their immigration status. "We welcome everyone at AltaMed and we are here to help them with primary care and their health concerns, providing quality care without exception," chief information officer Ray Lowe says. "At our core is social justice" (Kianickova, 2020).

Lowe teamed with the chief medical information officer, Dr. Lee, to launch their **digital transformational** journey. In order to do this, the duo set about developing a comprehensive plan that was rapid, agile, and included input from business stakeholders in clinical and financial operation areas (Kianickova, 2020). "A tech initiative without operational buy-in will not deliver the right outcomes," Lowe says. "I always keep in mind what the corresponding workflow is and what the [key performance indicators]

are that we need to meet for the organization, thinking not just in terms of technology, but from an operational perspective" (Kianickova, 2020).

"Digital transformation is not easy," he adds. "Aligning the organization requires flawless delivery of operations. Good IT requires detailed planning and strong operations to ensure the organization will be successful. Ultimately, I think IT needs to run like magic."

The last 2 years have certainly produced many benefits. AltaMed has hardened core services, implementing solutions for televisits, remote patient monitoring, patient portals, and social determinants of health. Key to their success has been the interprofessional relationship with operations and clinicians, establishing an end-to-end simulation lab to better understand the patient experience.

ESTABLISHING TELEHEALTH PROGRAMS IN CLINICAL PRACTICE

Modern practice must be bimodal. Practices must be capable of offering care in direct patient settings as well as virtual environments. Telehealth programs are unusually intricate as compared with traditional healthcare programs. Substantive telehealth programs are only developed by a small number of organizations, because there are significant factors that hinder the development of sustainable programs. Even in a postpandemic era, the telehealth boom that multiplied overnight has significantly retreated. Primary factors include the issues of skills (as few organizations have individuals with relative experience) and management (Latifi, 2011). Adding to this long-standing dilemma are regulations that limit telehealth across state lines and lack of sustained material reimbursement. Unwritten is the greatest barrier of all: the lack of organizational will to change and modify care management and patient throughput. Today, most telehealth practices simply overlay enhanced technical capabilities upon old processes. This leads to dissatisfaction by clinicians and patients alike. The higher the dissatisfaction, the greater the rejection of telehealth.

Over the last few years, different lessons have been learned about the evaluation and establishment of telehealth technologies and putting them into everyday practice. Assessment of technology and evaluation of programs are the major factors contributing toward the success of telehealth programs (Puskin et al., 2010). As healthcare professionals face demands for improved patient experience and deal with complex issues such as population health, rural health access, health inequity, and chronic disease management, telehealth is no longer optional; it is an emerging requirement for practice success. Combined, these issues and market forces put significant stress on health services.

Clearly, telehealth can play a vital role in addressing and mitigating the challenges and exploiting the opportunity.

STRATEGIES TO ESTABLISH CLINICAL TELEHEALTH

Telehealth programs are unlike other businesses and require proper planning and strategic measures. To establish a clinical telehealth program the healthcare organization should focus on the following strategies: interprofessional teamwork, culture and change management, technology deployment, training, agile operations, human-centered design, legal and regulatory considerations, business planning, marketing, and finally, performance monitoring.

Interprofessional Teamwork

The assessment from the Institute of Medicine shows that interprofessional education (IPE) plays a significant role in providing effective communication between patients and healthcare providers. IPE assumes that the patient's outcome will get better when healthcare providers from different fields work together. Positive changes were observed while using IPE telehealth case activities in which the students were put together with the physician assistant. The main purpose of the research of Begley et al. (2019) was to implement and analyze the case activities of interprofessional telehealth by integrating them in the Dispensing and Patient Care laboratory course of pharmacy skills. Their research concluded that real-time telehealth experience with the patients motivated further interprofessional teamwork. One of the main advantages of the telehealth program was that medical students from all over the United States participated in real-time IPE (Begley et al., 2019).

Interprofessional collaboration specifically while using televisits was described by Jarvis-Selinger et al. (2008). Telehealth

AAMC Telehealth Competencies Domain 3: Communication via Telehealth

Entering residency	Entering practice (recent residency graduate)	Experienced faculty physician (3–5 years post-residency)
3a. Explains how remote patients' social supports and healthcare providers can be incorporated into telehealth interactions and the care plan (e.g., asynchronous communication and the storage and forwarding of data)	3b. Determines situations in which patients' social supports and healthcare providers should be incorporated into telehealth interactions, with the patients' consent, to provide optimal care	3c. Role models and teaches how to incorporate patients' social supports into telehealth interactions, with the patients' consent, to provide optimal care

AAMC. (2021) *Telehealth competencies across the learning continuum.* AAMC New and Emerging Areas in Medicine Series. Washington, DC: AAMC.

care providers were positively enthusiastic for having interprofessional collaboration with the nurses, physicians, patients, and healthcare specialists. Even the remote practitioners were able to gain more experience, which enabled them to handle extreme situations improving clinical outcomes. This aligns with Domain 3c of the AAMC Telehealth Competencies.

The research conducted by Ishani et al. (2016) was in a controlled trial on patients with chronic kidney disease (CKD). They researched the telehealth interprofessional teams to determine whether the team were delivering feasible care and if the strategies implemented by the telehealth interprofessional workers had an impact on the patients' health outcomes. Studies in the past suggested that home monitoring of blood pressure could improve patients' health outcomes in CKD, but the results of telehealth interventions were unclear in the past. Ishani et al.(2016) conducted research on the interprofessional clinical team, where each intervention was reviewed by a nephrologist, nurse, social worker, pharmacy specialist, dietician, and telehealth technician to develop long and short-term objectives. In each case, interprofessional care was found to be superior.

Telehealth interprofessional teams were integrated in the rural emergency department for remote access to electronic intensive care unit (eICU). The study showed that having telehealth interprofessional teams improved clinical performance. Telehealth video carts were purchased to provide eICU to the people living in rural areas. Multiple interprofessional teams participated to provide healthcare where they also helped to form a social learning context. Establishing communication with the patient and healthcare team improved the patients' care and experience. Fig. 5.1 shows the usual and simulated flow of clinical information (Bond et al., 2019).

The hard work of interprofessional teams to establish the metrics that will determine overall success after creating specified goals is critical. Setting the telehealth program goals and expecting a positive outcome is critical as the progress of the interprofessional team will be highly dependent on the improved performance (Broderick & Lindeman, 2013).

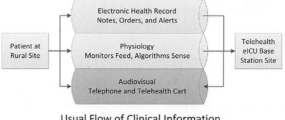

Usual Flow of Clinical Information

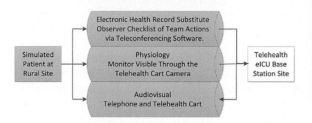

Simulated Flow of Clinical Information for Shared Awareness

Fig. 5.1 Schematic representation of usual and simulated flow of clinical information (Bond et al., 2019). (Source: Fig. 5.1. https://www.econstor.eu/bitstream/10419/190402/1/F2_1_Pereira-and-Fife.pdf)

Our work at the Cleveland Clinic in 2018 has proven the same. The move to interprofessional care helped improve patient outcomes and increased clinician and patient satisfaction. For all the evidence and experience, it remains clear that an interprofessional approach in telehealth programs is a key determinant of success. While we are seeing the emergence of virtualists (clinicians who specialize in telehealth), strong programs require a "team of teams" approach where every clinician involved in the treatment of a specific patient needs to collaborate closely. Team members include, but are not limited to, pharmacists, nurses, physicians, and medical technicians. It is now expected that physical or virtual rounds are attended by the full interprofessional team. Telehealth is a team sport.

Culture and Change Management

Technology is often the easiest of all the telehealth program building blocks. The most difficult key to programmatic success is culture and change management. Generally, culture is slow and even resistant to change. Telehealth specifically is disruptive to traditional models of care and organizational structure. An organization can have the most modern of telehealth capabilities but fail for lack of effective change management; conversely, problems associated with mediocre technology can be overcome with strong cultural capabilities. Culture and change management are considered soft skills and therefore easily undervalued or overlooked. However, the majority of telehealth and other healthcare technology failures are largely attributable to lack of change management.

One approach to ensure success is the use of Kotter's "eight steps for leading change" tool (Kotter, Inc., n.d.). Widely used over the last 20 years, the eight-step program has proven effective for ensuring cultural alignment and effective change management. The first step in this process is to create a sense of urgency and a compelling vision of why establishing a telehealth program is critical for the organization. The final step ends with institutionalizing change; in other words, making the changes permanent. You can adopt any program as long as it effectively addresses the cultural and change management challenges.

Technology Deployment

The integration of telehealth with other existing practice technologies gives new opportunities for lowering the cost of care, increasing care quality, and enhancing patient safety. Proper technology deployment will lead to improved experiences for all stakeholders.

Incorporating telehealth technology requires didactic and experienced telehealth education (Rutledge et al., 2017).

A telehealth program is a multinetwork program; therefore deploying the right technology is highly important. Every part of the fabric should be interoperable, deploying open standards such as application programming interface (API) and Fast Healthcare Interoperability Resources (FHIR) protocols. To ensure scalability and speed, cloud-based solutions are preferred. Patients' health data/records must be kept safe, especially as the magnitude of the telehealth program increases through a variety of modalities. Many telehealth programs require large investments, but this technology is worth the time, money, and effort; effective, modern technology will help save time and effort in telehealth programs (Puskin et al., 2010).

Leveraging telecommunication in telehealth technologies can help to build up health education and public health delivery. Telehealth technology has the ability to elevate the quality of healthcare with lower costs (Hsieh et al., 2015). This technology allows more frequent communication and regular monitoring of patients (Rutledge et al., 2017).

Minimum technical requirements need to be met when providing services for a telehealth program. Robust bandwidth is critical. Visual clarity is vital. It is estimated that 25% of the US population still have poor bandwidth or are without an adequate mobile device. This is particularly true in rural populations as well as in lower-income populations. High bandwidth is vital for telehealth services where communication is significant for essential care (Jarvis-Selinger et al., 2008). Every telehealth program must be bimodal and operate in both the physical and virtual spaces to accommodate all patients.

Training

A primary reason behind the slow uptake of telehealth is the lack of education and training. Research conducted by Lamb and Shea (2011) showed that healthcare professionals have limited skills and knowledge about effective telehealth. Without the requisite training, healthcare professionals are unable to encourage or assist patients with telehealth.

For education and training purposes, online education related to telehealth is considered the best practice. According to Edirippulige and Armfield (2016), online training is preferred because of its time-bending flexibility, which is advantageous for busy practitioners. In the post-pandemic era, remote, contactless telehealth training is the preferred option. Effective and efficient training for telehealth programs includes: (1) up-to-date communication technology; (2) advanced clinical technology; (3) training for the use of diagnostic devices on both the sending and the receiving end; and (4) access to technical support (Vander Werf, 2004). Many telehealth program failures can be attributed to lack of training and support. Avoid being penny wise and pound foolish; while the upfront investment is heavy in terms of time and resource, the long-term benefits pay for themselves.

Agile Operations

Healthcare organizations are trying hard to continuously upgrade their tools and technologies according to the latest trends. The main priority of healthcare organizations and healthcare professionals is to provide effective patient care that gives positive outcomes.

Implementing agile methods can help improve the effective implementation and development of telehealth programs. According to Fruhling et al. (2005), agile methodology is significant for telehealth technology development and focuses on the idea that coding and tools development should not be emphasized, but instead communication between the team members should play a greater role in project success;

in other words, talking often to your customer to ensure tele-health deliverables trumps technical aspects. Documentation is significant for developing software. Customer collaboration and effective communication are critical for the success of telehealth.

While most organizations will purchase turnkey telehealth solutions, some will build their own, and agile methodology is a key accelerator. Agile is more than programming; it is a new way of work. You want to avoid establishing a modern telehealth program on top of legacy operations. This is the perfect time to transform your operations to help enable telehealth program success. Key areas to discuss with the interprofessional team include operational workflow, primary care coverage, specialty expansion, and program leadership.

The final aspect of an agile operation is organizational structure. Simply adding a department of telehealth is suboptimal. You must consider a complete redesign of not just your operations but the practice structure. Organizational structure governs and defines internal operational components, major processes, reporting relationships, partnership arrangements, and external value chains. This structure allows the organization to quickly respond to changing dynamics, including competitors, customers, and the community. It is built to identify and respond to new threats and opportunities, enable differentiation in the marketplace, and determine strategic objectives. When new business opportunities present themselves, a resilient structure will allow for improved decision-making (Pereira & Fife, 2018). Having agile operations and a strong organizational structure ensures stability and enables growth.

Human-Centered Design

To increase the likelihood of adoption, satisfaction, and usability, workflows must be adjusted to allow the full incorporation of telehealth into traditional care. (Bhattacharyya et al., 2019; Kvedar et al., 2014). In human-centered design, impact to daily operations becomes central. It is wise to think through new processes to ensure compliance with novel telehealth programs. Interprofessional collaboration becomes key again as organizations must bring together clinicians, administrators, and experts in design to create new workflows. Many programs are suboptimized because they are additive to existing operations, leading to subpar results. Mixing telehealth visits with traditional models of care can lead to failure. Successful programs will take the time to design workflows, thinking in new ways to maximize the efficiency of both models to the extent that they will coexist. Mixing appointments between telehealth and in-office does not work well; asking patients to go through traditional methods of clinical access for telehealth appointments will lead to massive inefficiencies and dissatisfaction.

Creating internal simulation labs where new ideas and workflows can be tested will prove invaluable. Finally, mixing agile operations with human-centered design will help telehealth programs quickly modify approaches and workflow to minimize frustrations and maximize results.

Legal and Regulatory Requirements

Legal and regulatory requirements are constantly changing. There are many rules and regulations that telehealth programs must comply with. These include cybersecurity requirements, HIPAA, and strict billing protocols. It is important that you engage legal, compliance, finance, and risk professionals prior to embarking on your program. Additionally, as members of your broader interprofessional team, they should remain up to date on changes in these areas, as failure to comply with evolving statutes could have major operational implications.

Examples include the ability for telehealth providers to practice across state borders without specific state licensure, the ability to bill for televideo visits, and remote patient monitoring. Telehealth remains an evolving field, so appropriate due diligence is a requirement for sustainability.

Marketing

In the digital era, telehealth programs are best marketed through digital means. Digital marketing is a vast field that includes multiple platforms like applications, blogs, online ads, and social media. A big part of the patient experience is engagement, and it begins with marketing. Developing a systematic marketing plan is critical to promote clinical telehealth in an efficient manner. Dansky and Ajello (2015) stated that opportunities and risks can be pointed out with the help of strategic marketing management. A strategic marketing management approach is primarily future oriented (Dansky & Ajello, 2015) but also contains tactics for reaching customers in the present.

The 4-P marketing paradigm is the traditional strategy used for marketing, the four Ps being product, price, place, and promotion. However, traditional marketing strategies like 4-P do not apply as much in healthcare, because the service matters as much as the product. Dimmick and Burgiss (n.d.) stated that the four Rs (relevance, response, relationship, and results) are applied and emphasized in contemporary health marketing strategies.

Vander Werf (2004) mentioned three successful techniques that could help progress telehealth programs:
- Marketing to management: Ensure that practice management is informed of progress toward goals and the timing of each. In the event of obstacles, inform management at early stages with the solutions proposed to

solve those problems. Ask management for assistance whenever needed.

- Marketing to naysayers: Don't waste energy or resources attempting to persuade naysayers to your point of view. Try not to disregard them either. You cannot change your naysayers but you should be prepared to neutralize their impact should they impede program marketing efforts.
- Observations: Everybody wants to share in program success. Invite other members of your organization to be a part of your program success. Even those whose contributions were negligible should feel a sense of ownership.

Program Evaluation

It is critical to the success of the telehealth program to have baseline metrics established from the beginning and included in the business model. The evaluation should recognize the significance of nonstandard measures and the part they play in improving health and financial outcomes. The outcomes should include the measured patient experience and staff satisfaction; other evaluation criteria will be financial metrics and, more importantly, quality and patient safety benchmarks. Evaluation should occur while implementing the technology and at routine intervals after deployment (Broderick & Lindeman, 2013). Evaluation usually requires a small amount of funding and should not be left out of the budget process. Federal funding for telehealth programs normally comes with a component of evaluation, so you must include this as well (Puskin et al., 2010). Most federal funding requires evaluation of telehealth components including disease diagnosis, evaluation of clinical management, and clinical outcomes (Heinzelmann et al., 2005). Securing baseline measurements in every category will help you evaluate and guide the program to success.

Transparent reporting of such measurements and holding individual leaders accountable for the success of each component is a key criterion for sustainability and achievement of the business plan.

BUSINESS MODEL

For a telehealth program to be sustainable, it must have a functional business model. As described by Chen et al. (2013), the business model canvas comprises the following building blocks:

- Customer: Who are the target patients? What is the mix of existing patients versus newly acquired patients? How many of them would engage in a telehealth program?
- Proposed values: Agreed-upon values to help guide the program, especially when difficult decisions present themselves, requiring expedient responses.

- Channels: How will you reach your target patients?
- Relationship with customers: How will you ensure quality experiences? How will you ensure adequate engagement?
- Revenue streams: What are the streams of revenue by patient type? What is the growth potential? How do you ensure the success of your program without adversely impacting traditional models of care? What are the 1-, 3-, and 5-year financial projections?
- Key resources: Who are the key individuals and what are the required positions for success? How will you recruit these individuals?
- Key activities: What are the detailed steps and overall milestones for success? Who monitors the project plan, and what is the governance model?
- Key partnerships: Who are the key partners for the program? Who are the key vendors and provider organizations?
- Structure of cost: What is the total cost of ownership for the program (to include salaries)? How are variable costs monitored and contained?

In her research on telehealth programs in developing countries, Latifi (2004) cited a few other key capabilities that increase the odds of success. These include:

- Legal and regulatory framework: Most business models skip the legal and regulatory framework (which is why we discuss it in this chapter).
- Enforcement policies: Implementing telehealth in clinical practice will require some new policies and procedures to support enhanced workflows and expectations.
- Affordability and sustainability: The revenue model must be well determined and vetted by financial professionals.
- Manageability and sustainability risks: All risks must be identified with mitigation plans.
- Financial risks in particular should include detailed plans for multiple revenue streams.

It is vital to break down business cases and business models into components in order to understand and come up with scalable and sustainable telehealth programs. Dinesen et al. (2016) stated that business models must be developed in order for these programs to succeed. While there are limited business model examples in the literature, global interest in innovative telehealth business models has heightened (Dinesen et al., 2016). What these all have in common is a need for a financial proforma, which we cover in the next section.

Revenue Model

The revenue model is typically part of the business plan. We address it as an individual section just to highlight the importance of completing a reality-based proforma before embarking on a telehealth program. The revenue model addresses the appropriate pricing structure, revenue allocation among partners, and where return on investment (ROI) can be calculated. The costs associated with any new program, and the offsetting revenue, must be fully understood. This ensures a broad understanding among stakeholders and helps ensure the value proposition is identified and supported (Fife & Pereira, 2011). While the ROI for telehealth programs is more than just financial, the revenue model must be complete and measurable.

The circle in Fig. 5.2 shows the relationship between revenue model components and the elements that are driving the need of telehealth (Pereira, 2017). The VISOR model (value proposition, interface, service platform, organizing model, revenue model) is a basic framework you can adopt and adjust to fit your program.

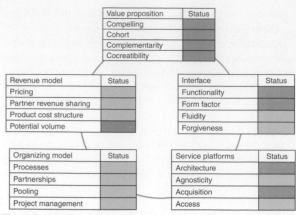

Fig. 5.2 VISOR model in the United States. (Pereira, F. (2017). Business models for telehealth in the US: Analyses and insights. *Smart Homecare Technology and TeleHealth, 4,* 13–29. https://doi.org/10.2147/shtt.s68090)

SUMMARY

Access to care continues to be an issue, and health equity remains a struggle. Consumerism demands multichannel healthcare. Technology is ubiquitous.

Modern practice must be a digital practice replete with telehealth program capabilities. Telehealth allows care to be delivered anyplace, anytime, anywhere, on any device. It increases patient and family engagement and enhances the overall clinical experience. Telehealth can improve the quality of care and increase patient satisfaction, and can deliver healthcare at more affordable costs.

Interprofessional teamwork is one of the keys to establishing telehealth programs in clinical practice. Telehealth is a multidisciplinary system, so it is inadvisable to hastily create a telehealth program in isolation; successful programs leverage the broader team in advancing telehealth objectives. While technology platforms are important, greater focus should be placed on culture and change management disciplines to ensure long-term sustainability.

A well-thought-through business plan with corresponding marketing and revenue modeling are additional keys to success. There needs to be attention and focus on achieving financial targets which are driven by performance metrics. These must be measured and monitored to ensure programmatic health. Enhanced strategies should be developed and executed to help meet all objectives.

Not to be overlooked, human-centered design principles and concepts should inform the emerging practice model and related processes. Avoid the temptation to simply replicate traditional models of care with telehealth technologies. While practices must continue bimodal care, telehealth should be operated differently, especially in terms of clinician and patient workflow. Not doing so is the greatest risk practices face when it comes to telehealth deployment.

In the postpandemic future, 91% of employers will offer telehealth as a benefit for employees, and the telehealth industry is expected to reach $55.6 billion by 2025 (Telehealth Market, 2020). The only way to solve many care access and care equity challenges is via sustainable telehealth practices. Every practice must deploy telehealth programs to survive. No matter how big or small your program may be, following the process steps outlined in this chapter will increase your probability of success.

KEY POINTS

- Successful telehealth programs include robust strategies around interprofessional teamwork, culture and change management, technology deployment, training, agile operations, human-centered design, legal and regulatory considerations, business planning, marketing, and performance monitoring.

- To ensure telehealth program adoption and sustainability, the design should be human centric and focus on the experience for patients, families, and clinicians.
- Strong telehealth programs are less concerned with specific technology platforms and more focused on culture and change management.

- For sustained growth, a robust business plan must be developed along with associated financial and clinical targets.

- Baseline measurements should be taken prior to the launch of novel telehealth programs so outcomes can be tracked and reported and adjustments made as needed.

❓ CRITICAL THINKING QUESTIONS

What are the key success factors for any telehealth program in clinical practice and why?

1. Why is human-centered design so important to patient, family, and clinician engagement and experience?
2. What are sample baseline metrics a practice might measure to determine the success of a telehealth program?
3. What are the basic components of a telehealth program business plan?
4. Name two or three reasons why every practice should deploy a telehealth program.

REFERENCES

Begley, K., O'Brien, K., Packard, K., et al. (2019). Impact of interprofessional telehealth case activities on students' perceptions of their collaborative care abilities. *American Journal of Pharmaceutical Education*, 83(4), 6880. https://doi.org/10.5688/ajpe6880.

Bhattacharyya, O., Mossman, K., Gustafsson, L., et al. (2019). Using human-centered design to build a digital health advisor for patients with complex needs: Persona and prototype development. *Journal of Medical Internet Research*, 21(5), e10318. https://doi.org/10.2196/10318.

Bond, W. F., Barker, L. T., Cooley, K. L., et al. (2019). A simple low-cost method to integrate telehealth interprofessional team members during in situ simulation. *Simulation in Healthcare*, 14(2), 129–136. https://doi.org/10.1097/SIH.0000000000000357.

Broderick, A., & Lindeman, D. (2013). *Case Studies in telehealth adoption scaling telehealth programs: Lessons from early adopters* (Vol. 1). Commonwealth Fund Pub. https://www.commonwealthfund.org/publications/case-study/2013/jan/scaling-telehealth-programs-lessons-early-adopters. [Accessed 01.11.21].

Chen, S., Cheng, A., & Mehta, K. (2013). A review of telemedicine business models. *Telemedicine and e-Health*, 19(4), 287–297. https://doi.org/10.1089/tmj.2012.0172.

Dansky, K. H., & Ajello, J. (2015). Marketing telehealth to align with strategy. *Journal of Healthcare Management*, 50(1), 19–30. https://doi.org/10.1097/00115514-200501000-00007.

Dimmick, S. L., & Burgiss, S. (n.d.) Marketing strategy for telehealth programs. Citeseerx.Ist.Psu.Edu. http://citeseerx.ist.psu.edu/viewdoc/download?-doi=10.1.1.197.9650&rep=rep1&type=pdf. [Accessed 10 October 2020]

Dinesen, B., Nonnecke, B., Lindeman, D., et al. (2016). Personalized telehealth in the future: A global research agenda. *Journal of Medical Internet Research*, 18(3), e53. https://doi.org/10.2196/jmir.5257.

Edirippulige, S., & Armfield, N. (2016). Education and training to support the use of clinical telehealth: A review of the literature. *Journal of Telemedicine and Telecare*, 23(2), 273–282. https://doi.org/10.1177/1357633x16632968.

Fife, E., & Pereira, F. (2011). Digital home health and mHealth: Prospects and challenges for adoption in the U.S. *2011 50th FITCE Congress - "ICT: Bridging an ever shifting digital divide,"* 1–11. https://doi.org/10.1109/FITCE.2011.6133431.

Fruhling, A., Tyser, K., & de Vreede, G.-J. (2005). Experiences with extreme programming in telehealth: Developing and implementing a biosecurity health care application. *Proceedings of the 38th Annual Hawaii International Conference on system Sciences, 151b*. https://doi.org/10.1109/HICSS.2005.257.

Heinzelmann, P. J., Williams, C. M., Lugn, N. E., et al. (2005). Clinical outcomes associated with telemedicine/telehealth. *Telemedicine Journal and e-Health*, 11(3), 329–347. https://doi.org/10.1089/tmj.2005.11.329.

Hsieh, H.-L., Tsai, C.-H., Chih, W.-H., et al. (2015). Factors affecting success of an integrated community-based telehealth system. *Technology and Health Care*, 23(Suppl. 2), S189–S196. https://doi.org/10.3233/THC-150953.

Ishani, A., Christopher, J., Palmer, D., et al. (2016). Telehealth by an interprofessional team in patients with CKD: A randomized controlled trial. *American Journal of Kidney Diseases*, 68(1), 41–49. https://doi.org/10.1053/j.ajkd.2016.01.018.

Jarvis-Selinger, S., Chan, E., Payne, R., et al. (2008). Clinical telehealth across the disciplines: Lessons learned. *Telemedicine Journal and e-Health*, 14(7), 720–725. https://doi.org/10.1089/tmj.2007.0108.

Kianickova, D. (2020). *AltaMed's digital healthcare transformation: Company Report: Healthcare global*. https://www.aamc.org/data-reports/report/telehealth-competencies. [Accessed 8 December 2021].

Kotter, Inc.(n.d.). *The 8-step process for leading change*. https://www.kotterinc.com/8-steps-process-for-leading-change/. [Accessed 1 November 2021].

Kvedar, J., Coye, M. J., & Everett, W. (2014). Connected health: A review of technologies and strategies to improve patient care with telemedicine and telehealth. *Health Affairs*, 33(2), 194–199. https://doi.org/10.1377/hlthaff.2013.0992.

Lamb, G. S., & Shea, K. (2011). Nursing education in telehealth. *Journal of Telemedicine and Telecare*, 12(2), 55–56. https://doi.org/10.1258/135763306776084437.

Latifi, R. (2004). *Establishing telemedicine in developing countries: From inception to implementation*. Amsterdam; Washington, DC: IOS Press.

Latifi, R. (2011). *Current principles and practices of telemedicine and e-health*. Amsterdam; Washington, DC: IOS Press.

Pereira, F. (2017). Business models for telehealth in the US: Analyses and insights. *Smart Homecare Technology and TeleHealth, 4*, 13–29. https://doi.org/10.2147/shtt.s68090.

Pereira, F., & Fife, E. (2018). A business model approach to realizing opportunities and overcoming barriers in e-Health. In *22nd Biennial Conference of the International telecommunications Society (ITS): Beyond the boundaries: Challenges for business, policy and society*. Seoul, Korea. https://www.econstor.eu/bitstream/10419/190402/1/F2_1_Pereira-and-Fife.pdf. [Accessed 1 November 2021].

Puskin, D. S., Cohen, Z., Ferguson, A. S., et al. (2010). Implementation and evaluation of telehealth tools and technologies. *Telemedicine Journal and e-Health, 16*(1), 96–102. https://doi.org/10.1089/tmj.2009.0182.

Rutledge, C. M., Kott, K., Schweickert, P. A., et al. (2017). Telehealth and eHealth in nurse practitioner training: Current perspectives. *Advances in Medical Education and Practice, 8*, 399–409. https://doi.org/10.2147/AMEP.S116071.

Telehealth Market. (2020). *Telehealth/telemedicine market by component (software & services, rpm, real-time), application (teleradiology, telestroke, teleICU), hardware (glucose meters), end-user (provider, payer, patient), delivery (on-premise, cloud) global forecast to 2025*. https://www.marketsandmarkets.com/Market-Reports/telehealth-market-201868927.html. [Accessed 1 November 2021].

Vander Werf, M. (2004). Ten critical steps for a successful telemedicine program. *Studies in Health Technology and Informatics, 104*, 60–68. https://www.amdtelemedicine.com/wp-content/uploads/2020/08/10_steps.pdf. [Accessed 1 November 2021].

Zieger, A. (2020). *Case study: One medical practice's experience transitioning to telemedicine*. https://www.hcalthcarcitto-day.com/2020/08/24/case-study-one-medical-practices-experience-transitioning-to-telemedicine/. [Accessed 1 November 2021].

6

Financing Telehealth

Leslie Haas, MBA

"If we don't reform how healthcare is delivered in this country, then we are not going to be able to get a handle on [the] escalating healthcare costs."

Barack Obama

OBJECTIVES

1. Describe why economics for virtual health differ from in-person care.
2. Identify the primary financial drivers for a clinician.
3. Outline the primary financial drivers for a provider organization.
4. Summarize the cost components of virtual health delivery.

CHAPTER OUTLINE

KEY TERMS

eConsult electronic consultations between two providers, typically initiated by a primary care provider to a specialist but sometimes conducted between two specialists

eVisit electronic visit initiated by a patient through which a clinical question is sent to a provider and response is delivered by message or email

Fee-for-service (FFS) the traditional payment model in the United States, through which providers are paid a predetermined rate, based on time spent or complexity, per service delivered

Payment parity when payors reimburse at the same rate for virtual services as they would for a comparable in-person visit

Provider a person or organization delivering healthcare services. Note: definitions for "healthcare provider" vary across the industry, but here we will use the broader definition, including not just physicians but any clinician or healthcare delivery system

Relative value unit (RVU) a unit of measurement, assigned by the Centers for Medicare and Medicaid Services to each service code, which is used to value the amount of time or complexity of each service. RVUs are used when reimbursing for services in a fee-for-service setting

Risk-based payments payment models predicated on prior per-patient healthcare costs and adjusted for relative population risk, to provide additional payment incentives to providers for lowering total costs of care and improving quality

ECONOMICS OF VIRTUAL HEALTH

In 2018 healthcare spend in the United States totaled $3.6 trillion, or 17.7% of the national gross domestic product (GDP) (Fig. 6.1). According to the Office of the Actuary in the Centers for Medicare and Medicaid Services (CMS), prior to the widespread infection of COVID-19, projections reflected over $11K of healthcare spend per person in the United States in 2018 (CMS, 2019). Given the impact of the pandemic, the spend per person may change significantly. Furthermore, healthcare costs continue to increase year over year, and according to the CMS are expected to continue to grow at 5.4% per year, which is faster than total GDP, and are expected to comprise nearly one-fifth of total United States spending by 2028 (CMS, 2020b). Although there are many causes for the high and growing healthcare costs, including aging populations and evolution of disease prevalence, this section will focus on a few of the primary reasons why costs for traditional, in-person care are high, and where telehealth can help to reduce these costs.

Supply and Demand are Local

One of the primary contributors toward high healthcare spend is that consumers of healthcare traditionally have been limited in care options to local providers. While patients in urban settings may seemingly have many options, given the higher number of health systems and clinics in urban areas, many of these providers operate at or above capacity and either do not accept new patients or have excessive wait times for appointments. Conversely, patients in rural areas typically have fewer clinicians within a reasonable travel distance, and the availability of these providers is quite variable. For these reasons, supply for healthcare services has traditionally been low, while demand is high, resulting in high prices for services.

Telehealth enables aggregation of both supply and demand for healthcare services nationwide. It allows providers to serve further geographies, thus enabling pooling of clinical resources, including physicians and other health professionals. For example, vendors like AmWell© and Teladoc© employ physicians from across the United States to serve patients nationwide. By creating large panels of providers and aggregating resources, these vendors are able to create staffing efficiencies, lowering the costs of delivering care and in turn allowing for lower price points to be offered.

Furthermore, with multiple direct-to-consumer telehealth offerings from telehealth vendors and health systems, there is greater supply of services available in the market, which creates competition to serve patients. These factors enable lower costs for:

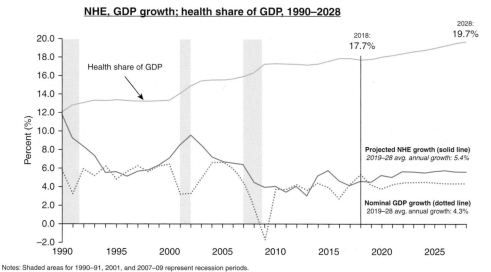

NHE, GDP growth; health share of GDP, 1990–2028

Notes: Shaded areas for 1990–91, 2001, and 2007–09 represent recession periods.

Fig. 6.1 Health share of GDP, 1990–2028. The national health expenditure (NHE) is growing faster than total gross domestic product (GDP). CMS. (2020a). *National health expenditure projections 2019-2028.*

- Health insurers: because of increased competition, insurers have greater negotiating leverage to contract for lower rates with providers.
- Consumers: patients are able to better shop for services, by comparing both costs and quality.

For these reasons, by aggregating supply and demand, telehealth is able to reduce total healthcare spend for services and increase the quantity of services delivered across the nation. See Fig. 6.2 for the relative impact of aggregating supply.

Scarcity of Specialty and Subspecialty Expertise

Across the United States, there are limited providers with specialty and subspecialty expertise. For example, in 2020 there were fewer than 13,000 oncologists across the United States, and only approximately 12% of oncologists were practicing in rural areas, leaving a majority of the US population with limited access to a general oncologist and even less access to subspecialists when needed (ASCO, 2020).

Whether for initial diagnosis, soliciting a second opinion, or executing upon treatment plans, patients typically have few options when seeking specialty care, particularly if they are in rural areas, and therefore are less price sensitive, driving up costs of care.

Virtual health programs, like eConsults and second opinion offerings, allow specialty and subspecialty expertise to be more accessible to providers and patients, at lower costs. For example, numerous second opinion offerings have been developed by health systems like Boston Children's© and Stanford Health Care©, as well as by vendors like Grand Rounds© and 2nd. MD©. These offerings allow patients from across the globe to solicit recommendations online from specialist experts for their diagnosis and treatment plan; this allows even patients in rural areas to ensure that the care plans developed are the best options. These offerings generate lower total costs in a few ways: (1) an online second opinion is often priced lower than an in-person visit; (2) patients save on travel and accommodation costs to visit specialists; (3) they allow specialized expertise to be more immediately accessible, ensuring patients get the right treatments sooner, rather than pursuing multiple ineffective options and driving up total costs; and (4) because care options are more "shoppable," more competitive pricing of services is encouraged. The AAMC Telehealth Domain 2 on Access and Equity may provide further insight on lessons of cost and access.

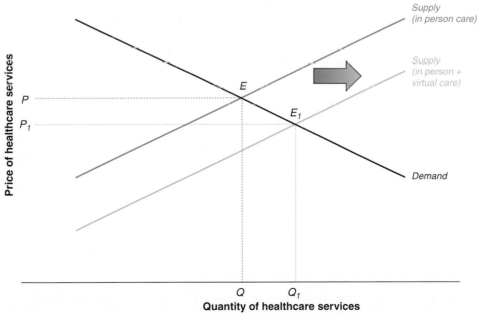

Economic impact of new telehealth services

Fig. 6.2 The directional impact of increased supply created by aggregating supply and demand.

AAMC Telehealth Competencies Domain 2: Access and Equity in Telehealth

Entering residency	Entering practice (recent residency graduate)	Experienced faculty physician (3–5 years post-residency)
3a. When considering telehealth, assesses the patient's needs, preferences, access to, and potential cultural, social, physical, cognitive, and linguistic and other communication barriers to technology use	3b. When considering telehealth, accommodates the patient's needs, preferences, and potential cultural, social, physical, cognitive, and linguistic and communication barriers to technology use	3c. When considering telehealth, role models how to advocate for improved access to it and accommodates the patient's needs, preferences, and potential cultural, social, physical, cognitive, and linguistic and communication barriers to technology use

AAMC. (2021). *Telehealth competencies across the learning continuum*. AAMC New and Emerging Areas in Medicine Series. Washington, DC: AAMC.

Transactional Versus Continuous Care

It is estimated that approximately 45% of US adults are unaware that they should have annual check-ups (Cigna, 2015). Further, a high proportion of patients only visit a healthcare provider when a specific health problem arises, often going to either urgent or emergent care settings, which tend to be more costly settings. For these reasons, healthcare has traditionally been quite transactional, and providers have not been well positioned to proactively manage patient health. This causes patients' conditions to escalate before being addressed and creates a higher total cost of care to treat them.

Because virtual health offerings typically require less from the patient to engage, including lower service cost, less travel, and reduced time commitment, they allow for increased engagement via more frequent, lighter touchpoints. Remote patient monitoring (RPM) is one example of a virtual health program that shifts care from transactional to continuous; by consistently monitoring specific health data (e.g., vitals, symptoms, outcomes, and activity) from patients when they are at home, clinicians may have better visibility into patient health and may more proactively address escalating conditions. By transforming healthcare from transactional to continuous engagement, virtual health may enable more patient interactions, better health outcomes, and ultimately lower total health spend.

FINANCIAL DRIVERS FOR CLINICIANS

In **fee-for-service (FFS)** models, billing clinicians tend to assess the value of services by the assigned **relative value units** (RVUs). However, there are unique financial benefits to consider when deciding what proportion of services should be delivered through telehealth versus in-person care. This section will focus on two of the primary financial drivers that may inform a clinician's decisions: productivity and downstream utilization.

Productivity

Providers, or billing clinicians, in the United States are largely reimbursed via the FFS model, which means a predetermined rate is paid to the provider by an insurer for patient healthcare services. In this model, physicians and billing clinicians are typically paid based on productivity, specifically measured by RVUs. This means providers get paid a rate that varies by service based on the relative amount of "work" required to deliver the service, as determined by CMS. Services like surgeries are assigned a higher number of RVUs than less complex or faster care such as office visits.

Some virtual services are reimbursed at parity, or at the same rate as the nearest equivalent in-person service. For example, most private payors, or commercial insurers, reimburse video visits at the same value as an in-person office visit of equal complexity; further, although CMS did not previously pay for video visits, during the public health emergency (PHE) for COVID-19, Medicare also began reimbursing at parity for video visits, although it is unclear whether or how Medicare will pay for video visits in the future.

CMS assigns other virtual services a lower number of RVUs than the nearest equivalent for in-person services, which means that providers get paid a lower amount for completing these services virtually. eConsults are one such example: CMS has assigned a value of 0.7 RVUs for an eConsult, but an in-person office visit, which is typically viewed as a comparable service, is valued at 1–4.6 RVUs for new patients, depending on the level of complexity of the visit.

However, the slightly lower reimbursement may be offset by an increase in productivity, given that the requirements to bill for virtual visits also differ from those for in-person visits. The time requirement to bill for an eConsult is only 5 minutes, whereas an in-person new patient visit requires a minimum visit duration of 10–60 minutes to bill for the services. If a clinician can complete two eConsults in 10 minutes at 0.7 RVUs each, or one new patient visit at 1 RVU, the physician's total productivity, or average RVUs produced per hour, will increase by conducting services virtually.

Downstream Utilization

Traditionally, clinic capacity is filled with a mix of low- and high-complexity cases, with little to no prioritization of patients based on need. Providers have little ability to escalate cases that have more urgent needs. Further, the majority of clinic slots are filled by patients utilizing clinician time and other resources to address minor care needs or questions, and paying providers at relatively lower rates.

However, through virtual care solutions, providers have the ability to manage low-complexity needs outside of the clinic and to triage or escalate patients requiring in-person care into the clinic, when needed. Continuing with the eConsults example, after a specialist has reviewed a patient's medical information and determined that the patient should come in person for further assessment or treatment, the downstream conversions typically have more complex needs and thus generate higher reimbursement. Further, a patient who receives a recommendation from a specialist to visit in person is much more likely to schedule and show up for the visit, rather than cancel or no-show, than those referred by a general practitioner. For example, a study at Stanford Health Care found that the cancellation rate for patients who scheduled a visit following an eConsult was only 11%, a reduction of 50% from the typical cancellation rate of 22% (Kim et al., 2018). For these reasons, the downstream conversions from virtual offerings provide additional value for the provider.

Exercise

To answer the following questions, assume that treatment times mirror the results from the Stanford Health Care eConsult pilot: 25 minutes for an office visit and 8 minutes for an eConsult.

1. Scenario 1: If a dermatologist works a 4-hour shift, how many patients could they typically visit in person? Round up to the nearest whole number. *~10*

CASE STUDY: STANFORD HEALTH CARE ECONSULTS PROGRAM

Stanford Health Care launched an eConsults program in 2015 in order to improve patient access to specialty expertise, care coordination, and clinical outcomes. Through this program, primary care providers submit a patient-specific clinical question to a dermatologist and receive recommendations for diagnosis and treatment options via an inbox message within the Epic electronic medical record software. Through this program, Stanford Health was able to deliver specialty expertise to, and enact care plans for, patients in an average of 16 hours rather than the average of 23 days that a patient would wait for a dermatology appointment (Kim et al., 2018).

Stanford Health found that 73% of eConsults were resolved virtually, and just 27% of patients were recommended to visit in person for further assessment or treatment (Kim et al, 2018). Further, dermatologists spent an average of 8 minutes to review and respond to an eConsult, which was a 68% reduction in specialist time required compared with the average 25 minutes for a dermatology office visit and completion of the required documentation. Further, cancellations for visits following eConsults were 50% lower than the average for in-person appointments, and both patient and physician experiences were positive (Kim et al, 2018).

Through this program, Stanford Health Care was able to extend specialty expertise more broadly and rapidly, ultimately reducing unnecessary specialty office visits and improving patient outcomes. Further, it was able to create new capacity for additional patients with complex specialty needs.

2. Scenario 2: If a dermatologist works a 4-hour shift, completing eConsults for 2 hours and seeing patients in person for 2 hours, how many encounters (eConsults + office visits) can they complete during the shift? Round up to the nearest whole number. *15+5=20*

3. If the provider gets credited for 0.7 RVUs for each eConsult and 1.5 RVUs for each office visit, do they get compensated more in scenario 1 or scenario 2? *In scenario 1, the physician is credited 15 RVUs and in scenario 2, they receive credit for 10.5+7.5=18 RVUs, so they are compensated more in scenario 2.*

FINANCIAL DRIVERS FOR A PROVIDER ORGANIZATION

Health systems and provider organizations have typically modeled the value of new offerings by assessing direct revenue and subtracting direct and indirect costs, to project profit margins. However, telehealth fundamentally changes care models, and therefore we must also evolve our valuation methodologies to reflect the new dynamics. In this section we will outline three of the primary financial drivers for a provider organization to consider when assessing telehealth solutions: cost avoidance, risk-based payments, and loss from downstream ancillaries.

Cost Avoidance

Healthcare delivery settings typically have very high cost structures to support in-person care. For example, physical space alone is expensive to establish and maintain; regulatory bodies have established standards for physical space requirements, equipment needed, and more that make medical spaces more expensive to maintain than many other buildings. As healthcare systems continue to expand their physical presence in order to attract and retain a broader patient population, the costs for physical space continue to grow. Further, dedicated administrative staff, medical assistants, supplies, and cleaning expenses are just a few of the costs that make in-person care expensive to deliver.

Virtual care eliminates the need for many of the components that drive up healthcare delivery costs. We will outline new incremental program costs for virtual care in the next section, but here we will focus on the costs that are no longer applicable for healthcare services as we shift care toward virtual modalities.

The greatest opportunity for a health system or provider organization to reduce costs is through reducing rent or purchase costs by using less physical space to deliver care. If one clinician begins working virtually on a part-time basis, there may likely be no reduction in the clinical space required. However, as whole departments or systems begin to adopt virtual care models, the physical space needed is reduced, as providers may rotate using shared clinical spaces.

Furthermore, as health systems or provider organizations continue to expand their presence to reach new patient populations, they will be better positioned to rent or purchase smaller, less expensive spaces, if space is needed at all.

Additionally, virtual solutions enable a reduction of additional support services like administrative or front-desk staff and cleaning services, also contributing toward a lower cost structure to deliver care. Some virtual offerings may even create efficiencies that allow for less support from medical assistants or nursing staff, by eliminating the need to room the patient and take vitals prior to the visit. Finally, virtual solutions support more effective triaging of patients to the right level of provider and care setting prior to in-person care, thus reducing unnecessary visits or rework for providers.

Risk-Based Payments

Traditionally, provider organizations in the United States have been reimbursed primarily in a FFS structure, which means they are paid more for delivering more services and paid at a higher rate for more complex services. However, provider organizations have begun absorbing more risk when contracting, and payments are shifting toward paying for value, rather than utilization. Through these risk-based models, provider organizations typically participate in shared savings, receiving a portion of the annual savings per patient, and get further incentives for improving the quality of care. In order to be effective in these payment models, delivery systems must find new ways to provide more effective care and prevent healthcare needs from escalating.

Virtual care evolves care models to focus more on patient engagement, preventative care, and outcomes improvement, which improves a provider's positioning for value-based contracting. For example, remote patient monitoring (RPM) allows providers to solicit consistent data points, such as activity tracking, vitals monitoring, or assessment of pain levels, to inform targeted interventions and improve treatment plans. The amount of effort for the patient to engage is fairly low, and so patients are typically willing to participate actively in health programs with remote monitoring. Further, by creating more visibility into the patient's health status when they are outside of the care delivery setting, providers can better customize and adapt treatment plans and intervene sooner, before conditions escalate.

By evolving care models to create more proactive and continuous care, virtual care models like RPM can help to position provider organizations more effectively to assume risk in contracting. By engaging patients through quicker, lower-priced encounters such as RPM check-ins, and replacing more costly encounters, providers can lower the total cost of care to serve patient needs, contributing toward shared savings. Further, by creating lower thresholds to engage and soliciting more visibility into patient health and behaviors, providers are better positioned to improve health outcomes, further contributing toward incentives from the risk-based payments.

Exercise

A health system launches a remote patient monitoring program and successfully improves health outcomes for patients from the baseline scenario (scenario 1) to scenario 2. To answer the following questions, assume the following data to be true:

CASE STUDY: OCHSNER HEALTH SYSTEM REMOTE PATIENT MONITORING PROGRAM

Ochsner Health System implemented a remote patient monitoring program for patients with hypertension to improve systolic blood pressure variability, with the goal of ultimately improving cardiovascular disease outcomes, all-cause hospitalizations, and mortality. The program enrolled over 800 patients with long-standing hypertension who had been under the care of a primary care physician for at least 1 year (Milani et al., 2020). Through this program, patients submitted blood pressure readings an average of three times per week, and clinicians would intervene, when needed, by adjusting medications or providing education or behavioral coaching.

In a 24-month period, Ochsner was able to reduce systolic blood pressure variability within this patient cohort by 23%. Patients were mapped to quartiles, based on their blood pressure levels from previous studies (<10.3, 10.3–12.7, 12.8–15.5, and ≥15.6 mm Hg). At baseline of the study, 30% of patients were in the lowest-risk quartile and 21% were in the highest-risk quartile; after 24 months in the program, 57% of the patients in this cohort were in the lowest-risk quartile, with only 12% in the highest (Milani et al., 2020).

Through this program, Ochsner Health System was able to show that RPM programs can significantly improve average systolic blood pressure for hypertensive patients. By better managing blood pressure, these patients will have reduced risks of cardiovascular disease, all-cause hospitalizations, and mortality (Milani et al., 2020).

1. Scenario 1: How much annual revenue, in FFS, does the health system receive at the baseline scenario? **$1,000,000**
2. Scenario 2: How much annual revenue, in FFS, does the health system receive? **$750,000**
3. If the health system participates in a shared savings model, through which it receives 50% of any total reduction in spend to manage the population, how much would the health system receive in total reimbursements? **50%*($250,000) + $750,000 = $875,000**
4. Now, let's assume that by improving population health outcomes and reducing avoidable emergency department visits, hospitalizations, and clinic visits, the system now has the capacity to manage 50 new patients, each bringing in new revenue of $5000 to the system. If adding this revenue to the total calculated in question 3, how much total annual revenue could the health system collect? **$250,000 + $875,000 = $1,125,000**

	First quartile (lowest risk)	Second quartile	Third quartile	Fourth quartile (highest risk)
Scenario 1: Number of Participants	100	100	100	100
Scenario 2: Number of Participants	200	100	50	50
Annual revenue (per patient) in fee-for-service to health system	$1000	$2000	$3000	$4000

Loss From Downstream Ancillaries

When a patient visits a healthcare provider in person, it is common that the clinician may either conduct a test in real time or place an order for a test to be completed at a nearby facility. Ancillary services, like blood or urine tests, are typically a significant contributor toward revenue generation for a provider.

However, during the PHE declared because of COVID-19, as providers shifted toward primarily virtual health modalities, health systems observed a significant reduction of ancillary services completed within the system. The total decrease of ancillary services during the PHE is speculated to have been caused by three factors:

- Clinicians recommended that patients wait for non-urgent tests in order to reduce the risk of exposure to COVID-19 by going in person for tests.
- Clinicians unintentionally ordered fewer ancillaries if the patient originated from a virtual offering.
- Because patients were completing visits virtually from home, ancillary services were also completed closer to home, at external testing sites, rather than within the health system.

At this time, it is unclear how much of a reduction of ancillaries will carry forward post-PHE, and what the resulting impact on health system financials will be. While the FFS model is most prevalent, this loss in downstream ancillaries may create a significant financial loss for providers. However, as systems shift toward more risk-based-contracting, a reduction in total ancillary orders, particularly for unnecessary tests, will position the system better to create shared savings.

PROGRAM COSTS FOR VIRTUAL HEALTH OFFERINGS

As we have learned thus far, virtual health evolves care models to create new value for clinicians and provider organizations. However, virtual health also incurs new program costs that should be considered as we assess the financial value of an offering. In this section we will highlight three primary cost drivers: hardware and software, marketing, and other labor costs.

Hardware and Software

Hardware and software costs are typically the most significant investments made toward digital health programs. A software platform, whether developed internally or supported by a vendor, is required to power any digital health offering. Sometimes providers may choose to use a different platform for each program to select the best option based on the individual program needs; this may be the case if there are specific, unique capabilities that the provider prioritizes. However, frequently providers will select one platform that can support multiple offerings to create synergies; by building upon one single platform, the organization can spread costs across multiple offerings while also creating better integration across programs.

Selection of hardware—like phones, laptops, and carts—may also be offering-specific, but providers will frequently aim to leverage existing devices when possible. For example, many offerings may be powered on top of mobile apps, so that consumers do not require new devices. Additionally, it is common to develop solutions that providers can access from work laptops or phones. However, some offerings, like RPM or cart-based solutions, do require customized devices, which adds to the cost structure of these programs.

It may be useful to review the AAMC competencies regarding Telehealth Technology here.

AAMC Telehealth Competencies Domain 5: Technology for Telehealth

Entering residency	Entering practice (recent residency graduate)	Experienced faculty physician (3–5 years post-residency)
1a. Explains equipment required for conducting care via telehealth at both originating and distant sites	1b. Identifies and is able to use the equipment needed for the intended service at both originating and distant sites	1c. Able to use, and teach others while using, equipment for the intended service at both originating and distant sites
2a. Explains limitations of and minimum requirements for local equipment, including common patient-owned devices	2b. Practices with a wide range of evidence-based technologies, including patient-owned devices, and understands limitations	2c. Role models and teaches how to incorporate emerging evidence-based technologies into practice, remaining responsive to the strengths and limitations of evolving applications of technology
3a. Explains the risk of technology failures and the need to respond to them	3b. Demonstrates how to troubleshoot basic technology failures and optimize settings with the technology being used	3c. Teaches others how to troubleshoot basic technology failures and optimize settings with the technology being used

AAMC. (2021). *Telehealth competencies across the learning continuum.* AAMC New and Emerging Areas in Medicine Series. Washington, DC: AAMC.

Marketing

Many virtual health solutions offer new entry points for patients, such as second opinion offerings, on-demand video visits, and **eVisits**. These offerings create value for providers because they provide a lower-cost initial touchpoint with the patient, and triage patient needs to the right settings when escalation or further assessment is needed. However, most patients do not know to seek out such options to initiate their care journey, and thus marketing is critical to educate them about options in advance of them initiating care. Without marketing, such offerings will have no utilization. For these reasons, most provider organizations invest heavily in marketing for virtual health programs.

Other Labor

In launching and managing digital health programs, many teams must participate to shape and sustain successful offerings. Following are just a few of the types of people who should be involved:

- Program management: Typically driven by an operations team or function, program management resources will provide oversight of the program to ensure that the programs track against identified performance metrics and financial targets.
- IT: Virtual health programs require IT resources to support platform and hardware selection or build, as well as ongoing technical support to ensure the solution performs effectively.
- Medical direction: In order to ensure new offerings are clinically relevant and provide value for patients, a medical director or clinical lead should advise toward program design and provide ongoing oversight.

SUMMARY

Healthcare spend in the United States is incredibly high and continues to rise year over year. This is partially because of a lack of access to the right types of care. However, virtual health can help to shift the economics of care delivery to ultimately improve health outcomes and reduce the total cost of care.

Furthermore, both clinicians and provider organizations should evolve the ways in which they assess the value of healthcare services in order to advance with the changing landscape. Rather than valuing new solutions simply based on expected revenue and traditional costs, there are a number of unique financial drivers that should be considered when valuing telehealth offerings. Clinicians should specifically consider the opportunity to increase total productivity and to optimize downstream utilization. Further, provider organizations should assess cost avoidance, risk-based payments, and the loss of downstream ancillaries.

Finally, there are also unique program costs associated with building and maintaining virtual health programs, including hardware and software, marketing, and other labor. These costs should be assessed holistically, along with the new financial drivers of telehealth solutions, to evolve valuation methodology to match the changing healthcare landscape.

⚡ CRITICAL THINKING EXERCISE

A health system is considering launching a new eVisits program to be offered to all established patients. What information would you need in order to assess the financial viability of the program?

REVIEW QUESTIONS

1. How can telehealth help to improve the economics of healthcare delivery? Select the option that is false.
   a. By aggregating supply and demand.
   b. **By reducing the number of physicians required to deliver care.**
   c. By transforming care from transactional to continuous.
2. By delivering virtual health services in fee-for-service, physicians can receive greater total compensation in the same amount of time by increasing _____ _____.
   Answer: Productivity
3. What costs typically comprise the largest portion of health system investments toward digital health?
   a. **Hardware and software.**
   b. Marketing.
   c. Other labor.

REFERENCES

ASCO. (2020). *State of cancer care in America.* https://www.asco.org/research-data/reports-studies/state-cancer-care-america.

Cigna. (2015). *Nearly half of insured US adults don't know they should have an annual check-up.* https://www.businesswire.com/news/home/20151209005332/en/Nearly-Half-of-Insured-U.S.-Adults-Dont-Know-They-Should-Have-an-Annual-Check-up.

CMS. (2019). *Historical national health expenditure data.* https://www.cms.gov/newsroom/press-releases/cms-office-actuary-releases-2018-national-health-expenditures.

CMS. (2020a). *National health expenditure projections 2019-2028.* www.cms.gov/files/document/national-health-expenditure-projections-2019-28.pdf.

CMS. (2020b). *National health expenditure projections 2019-2028.* www.cms.gov/files/document/nhe-projections-2019-2028-forecast-summary.pdf.

Kim, G., Afanasiev, O., O'Dell, C., et al. (2018). Implementation and evaluation of Stanford Health Care store-and-forward teledermatology consultation workflow built within an existing electronic health record system. *Journal of Telemedicine and Telecare, 26,* 1357633X1879980. https://doi.org/10.1177/1357633X18799805.

Milani, R. V., Wilt, J. K., Milani, A. R., et al. (2020). Digital management of hypertension improves systolic blood pressure variability. *The American Journal of Medicine, 133*(7), e355–e359. https://doi.org/10.1016/j.amjmed.2019.10.043.

7

Telehealth Technology

Elizabeth A. Krupinski, PhD

> *"There's no better policy in a society then pursuing health and safety of its people."*
>
> *Ralph Nader*

OBJECTIVES

1. Explain the equipment required for conducting care via telemedicine, including equipment at originating and distant sites.
2. Explain the limitations of and minimum requirements for local equipment, including common patient-owned devices.
3. Explain the risks of technology failures and need to respond to them.
4. Introduce the reader to key ergonomic and human factors aspects of telemedicine visits to optimize efficacy and efficiency.

CHAPTER OUTLINE

KEY TERMS

Human factors examination of social, psychological, biological, and physical components that inform the design, development, and operation of products and/or systems in order to optimize performance, user safety, and satisfaction with the ultimate goal of maximizing the benefits and the user experience

Real-time videoconferencing synchronous mode of providing healthcare services to patients (or provider to provider) using videoconferencing platforms

Store-and-forward asynchronous mode of transmitting medical and related data for healthcare consultations, such as remote monitoring data, EKG data, radiographic images, and visible light images (e.g., photographs)

INTRODUCTION

Telemedicine utilizes a variety of technologies, but the practice of telemedicine is far more than just the technology.

Choosing the right delivery platform and other equipment is obviously critical and must take into account a host of factors: what the intended clinical applications are, who the potential users are, how everything will integrate into the existing

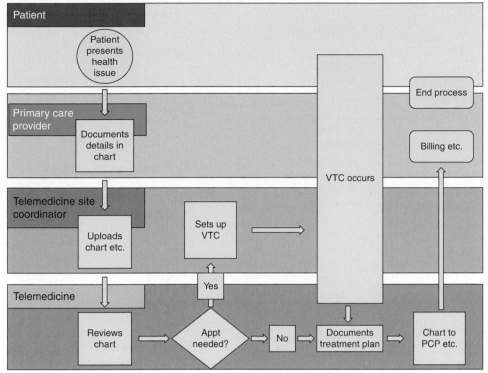

Fig. 7.1 Example workflow diagram of a telemedicine visit process. *PCP*, Primary care provider; *VTC*, video-conferencing.

technical and information infrastructure, and of course how much it will cost. However, once the choices are made, effective and efficient implementation is even more critical and requires a focus not only on the technology but on the users and their working environment as well. Creating a workflow diagram (Fig. 7.1) is a good way to visualize in advance of actual implementation what the various user roles are going to be, what technologies they will be using and what the steps will be throughout the telemedicine encounter.

Implementation of any new system, or even upgrading of an existing system, will require optimization of overall system performance and user well-being to maximize the likelihood of positive telemedicine experiences on the part of all users, including patients. In order to accomplish this, attention needs to focus on both the system (i.e., equipment, environment, processes, and procedures) and properly preparing user environments within the system. This chapter summarizes some of the fundamental aspects of both of these components and addresses the Association of American Medical Colleges (AAMC) Telehealth Competencies (Table 7.1).

AAMC Telehealth Competencies Domain 5: Technology		
Entering residency	**Entering practice (recent residency graduate)**	**Experienced faculty physician (3–5 years post-residency)**
1a. Explains equipment required for conducting care via telehealth at both originating and distant sites	1b. Identifies and is able to use the equipment needed for the intended service at both originating and distant sites	1c. Able to use, and teach others while using, equipment for the intended service at both originating and distant sites

Continued

AAMC Telehealth Competencies Domain 5: Technology—cont'd

Entering residency	Entering practice (recent residency graduate)	Experienced faculty physician (3–5 years post-residency)
2a. Explains limitations of and minimum requirements for local equipment, including common patient-owned devices	2b. Practices with a wide range of evidence-based technologies, including patient-owned devices, and understands limitations	2c. Role models and teaches how to incorporate emerging evidence-based technologies into practice, remaining responsive to the strengths and limitations of evolving applications of technology
3a. Explains the risk of technology failures and the need to respond to them	3b. Demonstrates how to troubleshoot basic technology failures and optimize settings with the technology being used	3c. Teaches others how to troubleshoot basic technology failures and optimize settings with the technology being used

AAMC. (2021). *Telehealth competencies across the learning continuum.* AAMC New and Emerging Areas in Medicine Series. Washington, DC: AAMC.

Domain 5 of the AAMC competencies has three skill areas, with the expectation of increasing skills from entering residency (recent medical school graduate) and entering practice (recent residency graduate) to becoming an experienced faculty physician (3–5 years post-residency). The first skill area concerns being able to explain the equipment required for conducting care via telehealth for both originating and distant sites. The second requires being able to explain limitations and minimum requirements for local equipment plus common patient-owned devices. The third requires being able to explain the risks of technology failures and the need to respond to them.

EQUIPMENT REQUIRED FOR CONDUCTING CARE VIA TELEMEDICINE

The equipment needed to start a telemedicine program is impacted by a variety of factors. Although cost is clearly a major consideration, it should not be the driving force behind technology choices. Likewise, the technology should also not be the driving force. Rather, the driving forces should be the system within which telemedicine is to be practiced, by whom, for what clinical applications, and for what patient populations. No two telemedicine practices will be exactly the same, but there are some basic questions that can be considered when trying to decide what technology to purchase (Box 7.1).

Once these types of core questions have been addressed, it is then possible to consider different technologies. A few basic categories form the basis of most telemedicine programs. Most of the basic technology requirements are the same for both the originating and referring sites, although certain clinical specialties and application areas (e.g., tele-ICU, tele-stroke, tele-cardiology) will require more dedicated equipment and different peripheral devices. The internet is clearly needed (although there are other less commonly used options, like satellite), and typical costs range from $50–$100/month for patients and solo practitioners to $500–$1500 for larger clinics and smaller hospitals, and higher amounts for larger hospital systems. Costs and quality will vary as a function of carrier, geography, and basic telecommunications infrastructure. Cellular options are also useful in some programs and typically cost the same as the internet. The minimum internet speed required (mainly with respect to videoconferencing) will actually vary as a function of the platform used. For most basic-option platforms (e.g., Zoom, Skype), minimum upload speeds range from 128 Kbps to 3.2 Mbps (HighSpeedInternet.com, 2021).

In addition to internet connectivity and security, there is the issue of bandwidth. Bandwidth is not speed but rather the volume of information that can be sent over a connection. However, the two are interdependent: more bandwidth (think of it as an increase in the diameter of a pipe) means more volume and thus allows for greater speed of information flow. Although bandwidth is important for many aspects of information flow in telemedicine, it is most visible to providers and patients during videoconferencing encounters. Low bandwidth can result in poor video quality (e.g., frozen or jittery images). The video can be turned off and audio only used, but that negatively impacts the visit. In most circumstances, basic business broadband at about 10–100 Mbps is sufficient for smaller practices. HealthIT.gov provides a very useful summary of

TABLE 7.1 AAMC Telemedicine Competency Domains, Descriptions, and Number of Skill Sets Covered

Domain	Description	Number of skill sets
Patient safety and appropriate use of telehealth	Understand when and why to use telehealth, assess patient readiness, patient safety, practice readiness, end user readiness	4
Data collection and assessment via telehealth	Obtain and manage clinical information via telehealth to ensure appropriate, high-quality care	3
Communication via telehealth	Effectively communicate with patients, families, caregivers, and healthcare team members using telehealth modalities; integrate transmission and receipt of information for effective knowledge transfer, professionalism, understanding within therapeutic relationship	3
Ethical practices and legal requirements for telehealth	Understand federal, state, and local facility practice requirements to meet minimal standards to deliver healthcare via telehealth; maintain patient privacy while minimizing risk to clinician and patient during telehealth encounters, while putting patient interest first and preserving or enhancing the doctor-patient relationship	4
Technology for telehealth	Have basic knowledge of the technology needed for delivery of high-quality telehealth services	3
Access and equity in telehealth	Understand telehealth delivery that addresses and mitigates cultural biases and physician bias for or against telehealth, accounts for physical and mental disabilities, non-health-related individual and community needs, and limitations to promote equitable access to care	3

Adapted from https://www.aamc.org/media/47796/download

BOX 7.1 Basic Questions to Consider Before Purchasing Telemedicine Equipment

- What type of institution(s) or practice(s) will be involved in the telemedicine service?
- How big is the institution(s) or practice(s)?
- How is the institution(s) or practice(s) staffed?
- What is the staff's knowledge base and skill regarding telemedicine?
- What is the geographic location(s) of the telemedicine service users?
- What specialties and/or services will be offered using telemedicine?
- What is the patient population(s) served using telemedicine?
- What is the delivery model—real-time-video, store-and-forward, or hybrid?
- What is the system model—clinic-to-clinic or direct-to-consumer?

recommended bandwidth for different types of providers and uses (HealthIT.gov, 2019). The larger the practice, the more bandwidth will be required (and naturally, the higher the cost).

The computing platform is important, and there are options available including smartphones, tablets, laptops, and desktop computers. Prices vary considerably, but for patients and solo providers good devices typically can be purchased for $300–$1000; for larger systems, it depends on the number of each type of device required and whether existing devices used for in-person care can be used for telemedicine as well. The faster the computer, the better the audio and video quality. Most smartphones have adequate processing speeds, as do most modern (post-2015) tablets, laptops, and desktop computers. In general, a minimum of 2 GB of RAM (random access memory) and a quad-core processor should be available in all clinical settings.

A good basic webcam is going to be required for most operations and can be purchased for $50–$100. A camera resolution of 1280 × 720 pixels should be considered the minimum in all clinical settings; however, the higher the resolution, the better the image quality. More complex cameras with capabilities like remote zoom, pan, and tilt are useful in many settings where the consulting site has the control so they can, for example, move the camera to track a patient's gait as they walk at the originating site. These cameras cost more but might be worth the investment depending on specialty exam needs.

A videoconferencing platform will be required for most operations, and the patient (for direct-to-consumer) will in nearly every circumstance use whatever platform the provider indicates, so there is typically no cost to them. Some platforms are free, but care needs to be taken to ensure they are compliant with the Health Insurance Portability and Accountability Act (HIPAA). A basic system without a HIPAA Business Associate Agreement (BAA) (US Department of Health & Human Services, 2019) and encryption costs about $50/month, while one with a HIPAA BAA for 10 users is about $2800/year. More advanced telemedicine platforms vary considerably, but low-end platforms that support an electronic medical record (EMR) and perhaps basic scheduling can cost $50–$100/month, or as high as $500–$5000/month with exam cameras and other peripherals. More advanced systems for larger organizations vary as a function of features, institution size, number of users, and so on, and can cost $1500–$250,000.

There are no set minimum requirements as these will depend on each individual user or organization, but as noted earlier, use case scenarios should be identified prior to investigating platform options. If the goal is to integrate a platform with an existing EMR, it is important to verify that the platform manufacturer has previously worked with or is willing to work with the EMR manufacturer to ensure seamless integration. This might require additional time and financial outlay. A useful free toolkit (with video explanations) regarding features to consider when selecting a platform is available from the National Telehealth Technology Assessment Resource Center (TTAC) (National Telehealth Technology Assessment Resource Center, n.d.). The site also includes comparative analyses of many major technology options from numerous manufacturers but does not make specific recommendations.

Peripheral devices will vary as a function of clinical specialty. For example, a dedicated exam camera (separate from the webcam; a device that has live video output and supports one-handed operation) is very useful for dermatology; prices range from $500 to $7500. High-definition cameras (720 pixels minimum) are better than standard cameras (640 × 480 pixels), and the higher the frame rate (the number of frames displayed per second), the better (frame rates can range from 24 to 72 frames/second for most cameras). Aside from resolution and frame rate, an important consideration from a human factors perspective is the size of the camera and its maneuverability, both of which can only be determined as a good fit by trying them out, for example at a trade show or conference.

Video otoscopes are useful for ear, nose, and throat (ENT) and primary care and cost $150–$7500 depending on type and quality. Most have real-time and store-and-forward (screen capture) capabilities. Some features to keep in mind when selecting a video otoscope are resolution, color fidelity, image size (both live and captured), overall image quality, and ease of manipulation and use. Electronic stethoscopes are useful for many specialties; prices range from $100 to $5000, but the devices sometimes require a monthly subscription. Electronic stethoscopes convert acoustic sound waves obtained through the chest piece into electronic signals transmitted through special circuitry and processed for optimal listening. Some come with software packages that can analyze the output to help identify and characterize heart and lung sounds; many come with earphones to reduce ambient noise levels. Dedicated telemedicine carts cost about $15,000 and a dedicated room display system about $10,000, and these are useful for using in hospital rooms with inpatients. Dedicated equipment for specialties like tele-stroke services and maternal-fetal monitoring systems varies considerably but can cost $50,000–$100,000.

Simply having these devices available at both the originating and consulting sites is only half of the equation. As many of them are not commonly used during in-person visits, it does take some amount of training at both ends to efficiently and effectively acquire patient data during a telemedicine encounter. It is very useful to engage all participants at both sites in training sessions prior to actual patient encounters. These training sessions should not simply be explanations of how the technology works but should allow all users to go through the actual steps required to collect data, using simulated patients or other volunteers. A provider at the consulting site should understand the technology and its capabilities, limitations, operational modes, and maneuverability options, so that they can guide someone at the originating site through an exam if necessary. This is especially true when the person in the room with the patient is not an experienced healthcare provider but a telepresenter who may or may not have an extensive healthcare background or knowledge of what signs and symptoms to look for. It is also useful to have the users serve as simulated patients so they can better understand the patient experience side of the encounter. If the patient is in a home environment, guiding a carer or family member through the steps required to acquire relevant patient data will certainly require some additional skill and knowledge.

Sources of data that are not considered peripheral devices per se because they are not approved by the FDA (US FDA, n.d.) include physiological remote monitoring technology and other devices that transmit, store, and communicate personal health data. These are increasingly being used by patients to collect health-related data. Typical devices include smart watches that monitor activity levels, heart rate monitors, EKG monitors, Bluetooth scales, and blood pressure monitors, but this list keeps growing. Some devices provide only raw data, while some manage remote data, assuming that healthcare professionals do not look at all the raw data but use data mining approaches, analytics, recommendations for data integrity, and workflows that support reviewing only data that is out of range for a patient. Some devices are paired with apps that help with data storage and transmission, while others require the patient to record the data.

There are some points to bear in mind with these types of devices. Patient-generated data are subject to the same security and privacy requirements as any other patient health information, whether the data are *requested* or *accepted* by the provider. Providers or their organizations should have a policy in place on how unsolicited patient data will be used, if at all, when presented by the patient prior to, during the course of, or after a visit. Providers or organizations that accept and use unsolicited patient-generated data for medical decision-making should keep the data as a part of the EMR or other health record storage systems; they should have a policy regarding the use of patient-generated data by consumer devices not considered medical devices, stating whether the data may be accepted. It is important for providers to research the devices and any independent data on the validity and reliability of the generated data, as the data may not be reliable and may negatively influence medical decisions. Metrics like sensitivity (proportion of true positives) and specificity (proportion of true negatives, the opposite of which is false positives or false alarms) are important to obtain, if possible, from the device manufacturer. It is also important to recognize that even if a device has data showing that it has good performance metrics, this may not be the case when it is used by real patients in the real world who may not be using it according to recommended procedures.

When considering technology options and vendors, it is important to consider the existing infrastructure, what is lacking, and what staff and staff time are going to be required to install any new technologies and get them operational. This cost could be minimal at the solo practitioner level, but at the level of larger systems could cost anywhere from $30,000 to $400,000 depending on the options required and systems involved (e.g., EMR, billing).

Staff training on the various technologies is critical and may incur some cost as well, depending on how it is provided and by whom.

Although an organization's IT team may be familiar with telemedicine in general, they may not have the in-depth knowledge required to help make effective decisions about what technologies to use under the variety of case scenarios involved in telemedicine. Thus it is useful to reach out to those who are familiar with telemedicine technology specifically. There are two key resources available to those interested. The first is TTAC (https://telehealth-technology.org/), which has a number of technology toolkits (e.g., Clinician's Guide to Video Platforms, mHealth App Selection, Patient Exam Cameras, Technology Assessment 101), an Innovation Watch, and a number of useful videos on technology selection; TTAC staff are also available for technical assistance and inquiries. The second is the National Consortium of Telehealth Resource Centers (NCTRC; https://www.telehealthresourcecenter.org/). There are 12 regional and 2 national telehealth resource centers (TRCs)—one of which is TTAC and the other the Center for Connected Health Policy, which provides up-to-date information about telehealth-related laws, regulations and Medicaid programs—that have been established to provide assistance, education, and information to organizations and individuals who are actively providing or interested in providing healthcare at a distance.

The TRCs are funded by cooperative agreements by the Office for the Advancement of Telehealth (OAT) within the Health Resources and Services Administration of the US Department of Health and Human Services which started in 2002. The TRCs provide technical assistance, generally at no cost, to telehealth stakeholders, including state and local healthcare facilities, healthcare administrators, chief financial officers, healthcare providers, and patients. They work collaboratively as the NCTRC.

RISKS OF TECHNOLOGY FAILURES AND THE NEED TO RESPOND TO THEM

The majority of major technology failures should be readily handled by an organization's IT team or the manufacturer of the equipment. Thus it is necessary to have in place processes and protocols for reporting failures, expectations for time to fix and return to operational status both internally (at originating and consulting sites) and externally. These expectations and organizational requirements should be clearly detailed in any contractual agreements.

There is little expectation that a provider or other telemedicine staff member will be able to fix a hardware or software malfunction or breakdown. They should be aware of the processes and protocols noted above for major issues. They should, however, be able to deal with some of the more common technical issues that arise which are less related to outright technology failure than to human factors and technology glitches, especially in the context of direct-to-consumer telemedicine.

Prior to any telemedicine encounter with a patient, especially the first encounter, it is necessary to educate the patient and set expectations. This can be done in a variety of ways, including sending them concise, easy-to-read information prior to the visit; providing a link to a short video explaining what telemedicine is and what to expect (there are quite a few available online); or having a scheduler, nurse, physician's assistant, or other staff member explain the process and technology. Part of this introduction should include information about technology security and privacy measures. It is best, especially with direct-to-consumer services, to use a platform that does not require any sort of download or special software, but rather simply requires the user to clink a link or use a similarly simple method to enter the visit. No matter what method is used, the provider should always start each visit with a brief recap and setting of expectations and an opportunity for the patient to ask questions.

The introduction and recap should include information about what to do in the case of a technology failure. For example, if the internet connection is lost but the visit is to continue by a phone call, who will call whom, at what number, and within what time frame. During the telemedicine visit the provider should be able to troubleshoot common technology problems, like those in Box 7.2.

> **BOX 7.2   Common Technology Problems and Functions Providers Should Be Able to Troubleshoot and Explain to Those on the Other Side of the Visit, Including Patients**
>
> - How to start a video camera and microphone
> - How to adjust video settings and speaker volume
> - How to position the camera
> - How to turn off the video in case of bandwidth issues
> - How to turn off the recording function if it is on
> - How to reboot a device and start again
> - How to check internet speed
> - How to enable Bluetooth on a device in order to upload data from a peripheral or other device
> - How to admit other care team members into the session
> - How to disable (then reenable) a firewall
> - How to screen share

DESIGNING TELEMEDICINE ENVIRONMENTS

There are several things to consider from a practical as well as a human factors point of view when designing or preparing a facility or room for telemedicine (Krupinski, 2014; Major, 2005). Special attention should be paid to special populations like elderly patients (Charness et al., 2012) or those with mobility, visual, hearing, or other challenges. Many telemedicine clinics are not going to be newly designed and built, but rather will be existing rooms converted for use as telemedicine rooms. These rooms may not have been used previously for clinical purposes but may have simply been a storage area cleared out for telemedicine use. Thus room design can be a challenge, but there are a few basic principles that will help to create a workable clinical space. As healthcare delivery changes (e.g., as a result of a global pandemic or other crisis), telemedicine visits may be conducted in even more diverse settings, but the same core principles can be applied to create a suitable environment. Although it is rarely possible to control the environment in the direct-to-patient model, many of these principles can be used to help patients understand some basic ideas that will enhance their experience (e.g., room lighting and camera placement).

Room Design

During the planning stages, it is useful to begin by measuring the space and drawing out a floor plan to indicate where lighting fixtures go, where doors and windows are, where air vents are, and so on. Having the people who are going to use the room think about and possibly act out the various scenarios that are likely to occur can also be helpful. For example, neurology clinics often see patients with mobility challenges, and a key part of many exams is an assessment of the patient's gait and ability to navigate from one location to another. A consulting neurologist may want to view the patient walking from one end of a room to the other using **real-time videoconferencing** (VTC) equipment. The clinic room therefore needs to be long enough to accommodate this walk, needs to be free of obstacles to avoid the patient tripping and falling, and if possible, needs to have room enough to accommodate walkers or wheelchairs. The neurologist may need to move the camera remotely to follow the patient, or the on-site healthcare provider may need to move the camera physically.

If a patient site is going to have a specific telemedicine clinic room to accommodate different clinical specialty visits, it will need to house real-time VTC equipment, store-and-forward equipment (e.g., digital camera), and peripheral devices (e.g., electronic stethoscope, digital ENT scope, ultrasound) along with the standard exam room equipment. The design depends on the room and the operation requirements, but at a minimum it typically needs to accommodate all the equipment and two people (the patient and the healthcare provider) comfortably. There should be a desk with a computer that will likely serve as the store-and-forward hub where images can be transferred from digital cameras, case records created, and data transmitted to the teleconsultant for interpretation. A phone should also be available in case an alternate means of communicating is required. The key is to have all the necessary equipment organized with easy reaching distance so there are no risks of injury trying to access and use it. Standard ergonomic concerns about monitor height, monitor distance, mouse placement, and task lighting should be dealt with to avoid user injuries (e.g., carpal tunnel, lower back issues) (Occupational Safety and Health Administration, n.d.).

Telemedicine rooms must not be too crowded with lots of equipment wires hanging loose or running along the floor. This is especially crucial with patients who may have mobility and stability problems. Those using a cane, walker, or wheelchair need to be able to enter the room and navigate safely without worrying about tripping on loose wires, bumping into furniture/equipment, or injuring themselves.

The geographic location of the room is also important. A room located near the outpatient check-in wing of a hospital or clinic will likely get a wide variety of cases referred to telemedicine simply by its proximity and familiarity. A room in the pediatric wing will yield more pediatric cases, but the overall practice may use telemedicine less because it is too difficult to send patients to a dedicated wing. One option is a dedicated telemedicine room with equipment that is portable and easy to manipulate so it can be transported to the patient. This is very feasible, for example, in dermatology, where the key piece of equipment is a digital camera. Most real-time VTC devices (i.e., carts) are quite portable and easily transported around hospitals and clinics for tele-consults.

Room and outside environments should also be considered. For example, in desert environments, fine dirt or dust from the outside can ruin equipment, while in humid environments, mold and mildew may be issues. Heat, cold, and humidity can be issues, so adequate heating and cooling systems with appropriate filters (e.g., dust) may be required. Patients must be protected as well as the equipment. If they are already not feeling well or are stressed by being in a hospital, they may react poorly if placed in a small hot room for even a short amount of time.

Lighting

Lighting needs to be considered carefully. Telemedicine rooms can serve many purposes (especially in home environments), so a single lighting system may not be adequate. When the room is serving as an office to work on patient records or other paperwork, standard office lighting for computer environments should be used (Krupinski, 2014; Major, 2005). Clinically, it is easier to establish a trusting relationship if the patient is comfortable and is not straining to see the healthcare provider. If the healthcare provider needs to show the patient something such as the label on a medication, the color of some pills, radiographic images, or some other data, it is important that the patient be able to clearly see the information so they can better comprehend it.

Some key points to consider include are summarized in Box 7.3.

BOX 7.3 Key Lighting Considerations for Telemedicine Encounters

- Avoid colored lighting (e.g., yellow)
- Artificial "natural" light is preferred
- 3200–4000 K is a warm, white light and is recommended
- Fluorescent lighting is preferred
  - Can use low-end 3500-K "home" fixtures but commercial 5000-K white light is better
  - Dedicated fixtures (e.g., indirect, wall fluorescent fixtures) are preferred for dedicated videoconferencing and are available in cool white to reduce ambient heating
- For digital photo acquisition, the room should be well lit (150 foot-candles) using white light, fluorescent daylight, or full-spectrum bulbs instead of incandescent bulbs

- For video-based visits the best lighting is 300–500 lux, angled away from participants to avoid shadows
  - Avoid downlighting as it creates facial shadows
  - To achieve vertical illumination on subjects, place and aim fixtures 35–40 degrees above horizontal
  - If using only one light source, place as close as possible, from the same direction as the camera but in back rather than in front of the camera
  - Using multiple frontal light helps improve perception of a "3D" image
  - Backlighting helps body stand out from background
  - Use desk lamp off to one side for task lighting and fill lighting to compensate for poor conditions
  - Avoid reflecting/glare surfaces in field of view

Once a real-time exam is taking place or digital images have been acquired for the telemedicine consult, the room lighting can be adjusted appropriately. The key is that the participants at both ends need to see each other clearly and the participants need to look as close to "normal" as possible with respect to skin tone and so on, because these are diagnostic encounters. Some types of lighting distort skin tones, and poor lighting angles cast shadows that can mask relevant clinical signs.

Optimizing the visual components of the telemedicine visit is in many ways more important than the visual experience of visiting a provider in person. In person, a provider has access to all of their senses when evaluating a patient, but in telemedicine they are limited to sight and sound. During telemedicine visits for some issues (e.g., mental/behavioral health), providers cannot smell the patient to determine, for example, whether they have been drinking alcohol or have not showered recently, so visual clues can become far more relevant.

Although haptic technologies are being developed for remote touch, currently it is not possible to palpate the patient or even reach over and give them a comforting pat on the arm. Even sight and sound are limited to some degree. For example, it may not be possible to see the patient's entire body, causing the clinician to miss subtle movements like a tapping foot indicating nervousness or anxiety. Sound systems may not permit full appreciation of changes in tone, volume, or tremors. Our sixth sense, which is so active when we are in close proximity to others, is muted in a telemedicine encounter, reducing to some extent our sense of presence or gut reactions to a patient's presentation. Being aware of these limitations and developing ways to extract information about patient status using the tools at hand is essential to a successful telemedicine visit.

> To learn more, read the chapter on overcoming these barriers with physical exam techniques

Reducing Distractions

The room background (e.g., walls, floors, windows) is critical as well. Light blue is the recommended color for telemedicine rooms, but it is recommended that one or two walls be painted blue, rather than the whole room. Light blue tends not to interfere or interact with most light spectrums (reducing distortions in skin color, for example) and it conveys a sense a calm and trust. This way the color temperature of the skin will not be affected during videoconferencing or still photo acquisition. Flat latex blue paint is preferred over gloss or semi-gloss to avoid glare and reflections (even though glossy paints are

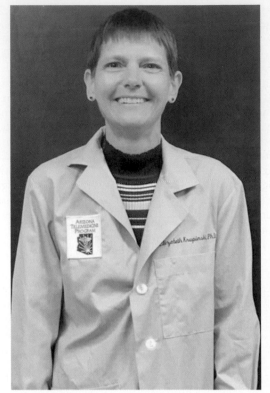

Fig. 7.2 Example of a blue telemedicine coat used to reduce glare during video-based telemedicine visits.

preferred in hospitals because they are easier to clean). Glare is especially difficult for older patients (and providers) who already have vision problems. Another source of glare is the traditional white lab coat, and thus it is recommended that a blue lab coat be worn instead (Fig. 7.2). If not wearing a lab coat, try to avoid flashy, busy clothes with lots of patterns and colors, and big, dangling jewelry. Participants should not face the camera with a window in the background; try to avoid windows altogether in the camera view, to reduce lighting problems and avoid privacy breaches.

It is also important to keep the view as uncluttered as possible on both sides of a real-time VTC meeting. From the patient's perspective, they should be able to focus on the provider without distracting details or objects in the background, and the provider needs to have an unobstructed view of the patient without a lot of clutter so they do not get distracted either. This can be difficult when the setting is the patient's home, but providing them with advance session instructions on how to create a good environment for a televisit can obviate many potential problems.

Sound

Sound is also an important factor for creating a successful visit. A quiet environment where neither party has loud background noise or the possibility to be interrupted is desirable. Speaker and microphone capabilities and placement are important and may need to be adjusted during the visit. Some patients are softly spoken or have trouble projecting, so the microphone needs to be placed close to them or the settings on the microphone adjusted. Either the speakers may have to be placed closer to them or the volume turned up so as to compensate for hearing loss or poor acoustics. It is important in all situations to ask the patient at the beginning of the visit if they are able to comfortably see and hear the provider, and to make adjustments if necessary. In particular, it is important to know in advance when setting up the visit whether patients (or providers) have disabilities that must be accommodated. There are a number of useful websites providing tips on how to accommodate visual and auditory disabilities (Google Meet Help, n.d.; Hadley, n.d.; Oregon Health and Science University Casey Eye Institute, 2020), and there are companies that provide sign language services with signers specifically trained for videoconferencing situations. Numerous platforms are increasingly incorporating real-time transcribing of audio to text.

Cameras

Cameras should be of as high a quality as possible and should be secured on a stable platform to avoid wobbling and shaking. Tablets and phones may need stands to stabilize them, and users should be encouraged not to walk around during the visit while holding their device. It is not uncommon to have users in their cars at the time of the visit; they should be strongly encouraged not to drive, and if the provider sees that the patient is driving, they may want to consider stopping the visit for safety reasons.

Cameras should be placed so the face is clearly visible to the other person in order to avoid chopping off the top of the head or yielding views where making eye contact is difficult (Fig. 7.3). This can be accomplished by placing the camera above the face by about 7 degrees of visual angle or less between it and the user. The initial viewing distance should be relatively close so that mainly the face and shoulders are visible. Having the camera too close may give the impression of invading the other person's private space. During a visit, it is useful to zoom out to capture more of the patient's movements and body language.

Some useful tips for preparing for real-time video-based telemedicine visit include:

- Use stands for tablets and phones so you are not looking down or moving.
- Test microphone and speakers before you start—consider using headphones.
- Check your video and look at yourself before connecting.
- Introduce everyone at the beginning of a session (especially if someone else is in the room, such as a trainee) and have the patient do so as well.
- Ensure you have a clean, work-appropriate background.
- Useful features to practice beforehand include: screen sharing, breakout rooms, chat, waiting rooms.
- Record only if necessary—note any recording to client and get their permission.
- Practice—do some fake sessions with different scenarios with colleagues!

Eye contact is critical during any social encounter but becomes even more important during a telemedicine visit, as it is fundamental to the REDE (relationship, establishment, development, engagement) model of patient-provider interaction (HealthIT.gov, 2019). It is a key component in helping to establish rapport and trust and allows for nonverbal cues in communication. In most cases and for most devices, the camera will be at the top of the device; thus it is necessary to periodically look up at the camera to give the other person the impression you are looking them in the eye. If you only look at the image of the other person, it is usually in the center of the screen, so you will not be making eye contact. Try to keep your head straight, as head angle and orientation affect the perception of gaze, and try to stay centered.

It is important to recognize that there is an etiquette associated with eye contact, as the "rules" for eye contact may differ according to a patient's culture, ethnicity, and gender. Certain mental health and vision conditions impact people's ability or willingness to make eye contact. Eye contact also changes with age, increasing from age 4 to 9 years, decreasing from 10 to 12, then increasing again through adulthood.

CONCLUSION

Telemedicine is not about the technology. The technologies involved are just tools to enable and improve the delivery of healthcare services. These tools need to be integrated efficiently and effectively into an existing or a new telemedicine practice, and processes and procedures need to be in place to optimize telemedicine visits. Adherence to human factors principles regarding technology optimization, environment design, and ergonomics can facilitate the transition from in-person to telemedicine care and reduce resistance and stress, making the experience beneficial and pleasant for patients and providers alike.

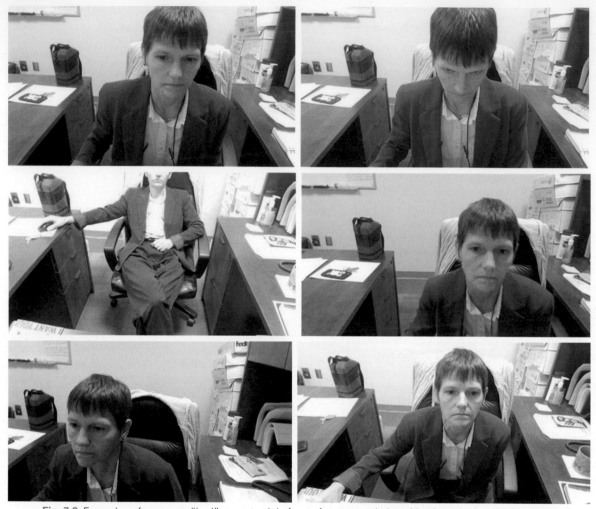

Fig. 7.3 Examples of common "bad" ways to sit in front of a camera during video-based telemedicine visits.

KEY POINTS

- In system optimization, consider the entire ecosystem that encompasses healthcare providers, patients, technology, and the environments within which they exist.
- Many professional societies have established minimum technical requirements for technologies used during telehealth encounters, thus they should be referred to when setting up a telehealth practice.
- Even if a device or app has data showing that it has good performance metrics, this may not be the case when used by real patients in the real world who may not be using them properly and according to recommended procedures.
- Having standard operating procedures and workflows in place for all aspects of a telemedicine encounter from initial scheduling through final resolution is critical to telemedicine success.

CRITICAL THINKING EXERCISE

1. In your current telemedicine practice, are technological or human failures more prevalent? Why and how can they be fixed?
2. What steps can you take to increase situational awareness during a telemedicine encounter in order to optimize the diagnostic decision-making process?
3. Do you have a game plan and/or standard operating procedures for every aspect of the telemedicine encounter? How does it differ from a typical in-person encounter?

REFERENCES

AAMC. (2021). *Telehealth competencies across the learning continuum. AAMC New and Emerging Areas in Medicine Series.* Washington, DC: AAMC.

Charness, N., Demiris, G., & Krupinski, E. (2012). *Designing telemedicine for an aging population: A human factors perspective.* Boca Raton, FL: CRC Press.

Google Meet Help. (n.d.). *Google Meet accessibility.* https://support.google.com/meet/answer/7313544?hl=en. [Accessed 1 November 2021].

Hadley. (n.d.). *Low vision and hearing resources.* https://hadley.edu/learn?topic_id=14. [Accessed 1 November 2021].

HealthIT.gov. (2019, September 10). *What is the recommended bandwidth for different types of health care providers?* https://www.healthit.gov/faq/what-recommended-bandwidth-different-types-health-care-providers. [Accessed 1 November 2021].

HighSpeedInternet.com. (2021, August 2). *How much internet speed you need to work from home.* https://www.highspeed-internet.com/resources/how-much-internet-speed-to-work-from-home#video. [Accessed 1 November 2021].

Krupinski, E. A. (2014). Telemedicine workplace environments: designing for success. *Healthcare (Basel, Switzerland), 2*(1), 115–122. https://doi.org/10.3390/healthcare2010115.

Major, J. (2005). Telemedicine room design. *Journal of Telemedicine and Telecare, 11*(1), 10–14. https://doi.org/10.1177/1357633X0501100103.

National Telehealth Technology Assessment Resource Center. (n.d.). *Clinician's guide to video platforms.* https://telehealth-technology.org/toolkit/clinicians-guide-to-video-platforms/. [Accessed 1 November 2021].

Occupational Safety & Health Administration. (n.d.). *Computer workstations eTool.* http://www.osha.gov/SLTC/etools/computerworkstations/. [Accessed 1 November 2021].

Oregon Health & Science University Casey Eye Institute. (2020, May 6). *Navigating COVID-19 with a visual impairment.* https://www.ohsu.edu/casey-eye-institute/navigating-covid-19-visual-impairment. [Accessed 1 November 2021].

US Department of Health & Human Services. (2019, May 24). *Business associates.* https://www.hhs.gov/hipaa/for-professionals/privacy/guidance/business-associates/index.html. [Accessed 1 November 2021].

US Food and Drug Administration. (n.d.). *Medical Devices.* https://www.fda.gov/industry/regulated-products/medical-device-overview. Retrieved December 16, 2020.

8

Implementing Telehealth Technologies

Yauheni Solad, MD, MHS, MBA

OBJECTIVES

1. Understand how technology can be incorporated into the clinical process to provide care for a diverse group of patients.
2. Identify and explain key elements in designing technology-enabled telemedicine programs.
3. Understand and explain minimal technology requirements and technology-related limitations related to telehealth.
4. Explain how to approach the evaluation, planning, and implementation of a telemedicine program.
5. Understand the risks of technology failure, be able to plan for accessible technical support, and be able to understand and provide basic troubleshooting.

CHAPTER OUTLINE

KEY TERMS

Actor a type of user that interacts with the system

Clinical encounter a point in time when the professional transaction between clinician and patient happens, when decisions about diagnosis and treatments are made, and during which caring takes place

Cloud (or **cloud computing**) on-demand availability of critical IT infrastructure without active management by the user

Digitally enabled patient a patient that possesses both the required technology and the knowledge to participate in telehealth activity effectively

Distant site a site where a provider of healthcare services is located while providing these services via a telecommunications system

eConsult an asynchronous consultation program that provides an assessment and management service

Infrastructure a set of facilities and systems to support software applications and network components

Needs assessment a systematic process for determining and addressing needs ("gaps") between the current and desired ("wants") states

Origination site a site where a patient is located at the time healthcare services are provided via a telecommunications system, or where the asynchronous store-and-forward service originates

Process a set of interrelated activities and actions performed to achieve a specified result

Use case a written description of ways in which actors can use the target system

Video visit two-way, real-time video communication

Workflow a repeatable pattern of activity, enabled by the systematic organization of resources into processes that provide services or information output

INTRODUCTION

The rapid adoption of telehealth during the COVID-19 pandemic demonstrated the growing need for professionals proficient in telehealth clinical and technical aspects (Canfield & Galvin, 2018; Greenhalgh et al., 2020; Hollander & Carr, 2020; Ohannessian et al., 2020). This growing demand creates opportunities for a new group of domain experts to combine their understanding of clinical **workflows** with the fundamental approaches to technology implementation to guide the rapid development and administration of the new telehealth programs (Aziz et al., 2020).

Telehealth is a field of rapid innovation. Powered by the improvement in consumer electronics, growth in the adoption of artificial intelligence, and broader access to high-bandwidth networks, the telehealth role is growing across all medical specialties (Aziz et al., 2020; Connolly et al., 2021; Thomas et al., 2020). For every clinical need, several telemedicine approaches can be implemented. For example, real-time telemedicine visits (face-to-face video) or asynchronous **eConsults** can be used interchangeably for low-acuity clinical visits for chronic disease management of **digitally enabled patients** (Bashshur et al., 2014; Jones et al., 2014; Salisbury et al., 2015; Wootton, 2012). In most cases, technology selection will be guided by a combination of clinical needs, available **infrastructure,** and clinical workflow (Celler et al., 2003; Criner et al., 2015; Darkins et al., 2008). Overall, specific clinical needs that determine telemedicine **use cases,** combined with unique practice environments, should define the telemedicine technology selection (Criner et al., 2015; Najafi et al., 2021).

This chapter will review how to approach telehealth technology, from the general mindset of technology selection to crucial privacy and security considerations. We will discuss approaches to identify and select proper technology, guide technology implementation, and provide basic troubleshooting. Lastly, we will touch upon how to properly assess your risks and create robust governance structures to ensure your telemedicine project's success.

Domain 5 of the AAMC Telehealth Competencies will be reviewed in this chapter.

AAMC Telehealth Competencies Domain 5: Technology		
Entering residency	**Entering practice (recent residency graduate)**	**Experienced faculty physician (3–5 years post-residency)**
1a. Explains equipment required for conducting care via telehealth at both originating and distant sites	**1b.** Identifies and is able to use the equipment needed for the intended service at both originating and distant sites	**1c.** Able to use, and teach others while using, equipment for the intended service at both originating and distant sites
2a. Explains limitations of and minimum requirements for local equipment, including common patient-owned devices	**2b.** Practices with a wide range of evidence-based technologies, including patient-owned devices, and understands limitations	**2c.** Role models and teaches how to incorporate emerging evidence-based technologies into practice, remaining responsive to the strengths and limitations of evolving applications of technology
3a. Explains the risk of technology failures and the need to respond to them	**3b.** Demonstrates how to troubleshoot basic technology failures and optimize settings with the technology being used	**3c.** Teaches others how to troubleshoot basic technology failures and optimize settings with the technology being used

AAMC. (2021). *Telehealth competencies across the learning continuum.* AAMC New and Emerging Areas in Medicine Series. Washington, DC: AAMC.

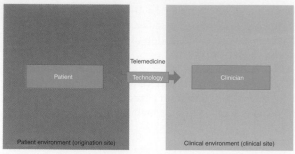

Fig. 8.1 Connective role of telehealth technology, as bridge between clinical and patient environments.

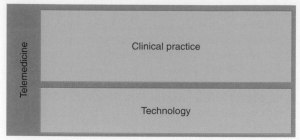

Fig. 8.2 Combined scope of telemedicine as a discipline. Neither clinical practice nor technology can be practiced or studied in isolation.

WHY DO WE NEED TECHNOLOGY?

This chapter refers to "technology" as a combination of tools and equipment used to deliver clinical care via telemedicine (Bashsur, 1995; Craig & Patterson, 2005; Perednia & Allen, 1995). In its essence, telemedicine is a technology-enabled **clinical encounter** that allows remote **actors**—in its simplest, form patient and clinician—to exchange clinical information to deliver care (Hailey et al., 2002; Sood et al., 2007) (Fig. 8.1). Overall, telemedicine is not a new idea, and its adoption is tightly connected to the growing maturity of communication technologies (Bashsur, 1995; Grundy et al., 1977). From the early examples of remote consultation powered by telephone to a modern surgical virtual presence, telemedicine technology extended clinicians' reach with the help of one or several communication channels (Grundy, et al., 1977, 1982; Lovett & Bashshur, 1979).

This tight connection between telemedicine and related technology makes it susceptible to the limitations of a specific communication channel. For example, in early 2000, one of the leading telemedicine technology vendors had to provide a high-speed internet connection line as a part of a telemedicine equipment deal. High-speed internet was still a novelty, and most hospitals did not have it. A high-resolution **video visit** can only be provided in a setting of adequate internet connection speed, and the inclusion of a high-speed internet line was a smart move to ensure that telemedicine equipment met clinical care needs.

It is important to understand that even though technology plays a foundational role in telemedicine, telemedicine is more than just technology—it is a combination of technology and clinical practice (Fig. 8.2). We need technology to power and expand our ability to provide care *when* and *where* patients need it.

THE FOUNDATIONAL ROLE OF TECHNOLOGY IN TELEHEALTH PRACTICE

The role of technology is to help establish a communication channel between patient and clinician. This communication channel is powered by a deployed technology infrastructure. Technology infrastructure includes all the equipment and local and **cloud**-based software that make telemedicine encounters possible. A patient location represents the **origination site** (Duncan, 1995). The origination site not only determines the applicable law and regulations but defines limitations on types of technology that can be used to provide a clinical encounter (Newton, 2014; Nittari et al., 2020; Stanberry, 2006). Direct-to-patient clinical encounters are mostly powered by a consumer-grade technology that is available at the patient location (Elliott & Yopes, 2019; Resneck et al., 2016; Uscher-Pines et al., 2016). Inpatient or ambulatory clinician-to-clinician video consults can have dedicated professional telemedicine equipment to support a higher video and audio quality (Vilendrer et al., 2020).

Both the physical location and availability of the deployed technology determine the functional capabilities of a telemedicine encounter (Holden & Dew, 2008; Pollard & LePage, 2001). Every type of communication channel comes with technical limitations that define what clinical activities can be reliably performed via this channel (Mohamed & Rubino, 2002; Seufert et al., 2014).

For example, both store-and-forward clinical consults (eConsults) and face-to-face video visits (telemedicine visits) may be an appropriate channel for nonurgent dermatological consults. However, variability in image quality, as a function of both a video camera and an internet connection, makes the consistent acquisition of high-resolution images challenging. Depending on the type of visit, specific communication channel limitations can impact the clinician's ability to perform telemedicine visits effectively. A video visit for a dermatology consult in a setting of low-speed internet connection may not be the best choice, and an asynchronous store-and-forward eConsult, with its ability to upload and share static images, may provide a better experience for both patient and clinician (Fogel et al., 2017; Liddy et al., 2019). Here, technology does not define the clinical practice per se because the dermatologist performs a regular diagnostic activity based on the clinical presentation, but helps to select an appropriate technology solution to provide clinical care. Understanding the limitations of synchronous telemedicine visits helped define an optimal store-and-forward eConsult clinical workflow that should be implemented to conduct dermatology clinical encounters in this particular clinical setting (Eedy & Wootton, 2001; Perednia & Brown, 1995; Warshaw et al., 2011). Eedy & Wootton, 2001 AAMC; 2021.

Why the Patient Should Be in the Center of Innovation

As discussed earlier, in its essence, telemedicine is an extension of traditional care that uses technology-powered communication channels to facilitate information exchange (Sood et al., 2007). Every clinical encounter, both in person and remote, consists of the following elements:
1. data gathering—for example, review of the past medical information, history of present illness, and physical examination;
2. clinical decision-making;
3. clinical recommendation and communication of the treatment plan.

Technology-enabled remote care can move any element of the encounter to a different channel (for example, data gathering from an in-person to a telephone or video visit) or a different time (asynchronous communication via secure messaging vs. synchronous communication via face-to-face video call).

Properly designed and implemented telemedicine technology should not disturb the traditional clinical practice but instead augment it by bringing care closer to patients (De Bustos et al., 2009; Hailey et al., 2002; Laxminarayan & Istepanian, 2000). Unfortunately, this is not always the case, and poorly designed or implemented telemedicine programs can decrease care quality, lower satisfaction, and even lead to technology-based discrimination (Hailey et al., 2002). These problems are usually the result of a fragmentation of the clinical experience caused by inefficient workflow design or poor technological fit. During all telemedicine program design stages, it is crucial not to forget that patients should be at the

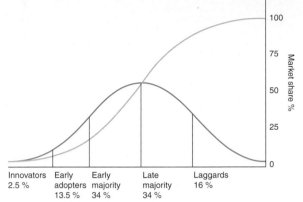

Fig. 8.3 The diffusion of innovations according to Rogers. With successive groups of consumers adopting the new technology (shown in blue), its market share light blue will eventually reach the saturation level. The blue curve is broken into sections of adopters. (Adopted from: Rogers Everett - Based on Rogers, E. (1962) Diffusion of innovations. Free Press, London, NY, United States)

center of innovation. Technology should enable care, not be the telemedicine program's primary focus (Chaudoir et al., 2013).

Diffusion of innovation

Telemedicine program success is only possible if the selected technology is well tested and adopted by target users. Luckily, innovation and technology adoption move in predictable patterns (Barao, 1992; Karahanna et al., 1999; Straub, 2009). When designing a new program, it is crucial to understand where the target technology lies according to the Gartner Hype Cycle (Dedehayir & Steinert, 2016; O'Leary, 2008) and technology adoption lifecycle (Van Lente et al., 2013). Now, let's discuss that in more detail.

In 1962 Everett Rogers proposed the theory of diffusion of innovation (Rogers, 2010). According to this theory, each innovation goes through predictable adoption steps from innovators and early adopters to laggards (Fig. 8.3). These stages are related to an adoption rate (the total number of new users who adopt new technology) and help innovators pick the right time (adoption stage) to introduce new technology. Successful telemedicine programs can be developed at any stage of technology adoption, but the level of technical and infrastructure support that should accompany the program deployment will significantly depend on technology availability. Programs deployed to the general public require a broad adoption of all critical components required for a successful

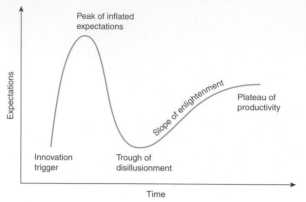

Fig. 8.4 Gartner Hype Cycle. (Source: https://www.gartner.com/en/research/methodologies/gartner-hype-cycle)

telemedicine encounter. Given the focus on wide adoption, the earliest most telemedicine programs should be introduced would be at the early majority stage. Ideally, a clinical program for the general public should be started when the technology reaches the late majority or even laggards stage.

Gartner's Hype Cycle is a branded graphic representation that demonstrates the maturity, adoption, and application of a particular technology (Linden & Fenn, 2003). Despite having a "cycle" in its name, it is unclear whether it is an actual cycle or just a graphical representation of a public's attitude toward a particular technology. Despite all the controversies, Gartner's Hype Cycle helps adopters evaluate a particular technology's readiness for broad implementation. The cycle starts at an "innovation trigger," which quickly leads to a "peak of inflated expectations" (Fig. 8.4). The disjunction between expectations and technological output is extremely important, because most innovators tend to "fall in love" with a new technology before it is ready for prime time. This disconnect between the vision and the reality is represented in the graph by a "trough of disillusionment." During this phase, all the downsides for the technology adoptions become visible.

A telemedicine program primed for widespread adoption should be based on a technology entering the "plateau of productivity" (Cranen et al., 2011; Peters et al., 2015). Interestingly, combining both graphs demonstrates that a "plateau of productivity" can only be achieved when the late majority is ready to adopt a particular technology (Van Dyk, 2013). This point is critical to remember, because it helps to select a mature technology that is ready for adoption when it's widespread enough to ensure the adoption (Fig. 8.5).

THINKING BEYOND INDIVIDUAL TECHNOLOGY

The approaches described earlier can help predict the adoption of a specific system, but when assessing target patients and their environment, a clinical innovator should go broad and assess the maturity of *all* related technologies that play a critical role in the project (Harst et al., 2019; Miller, 2003).

For example, the adoption of smartphone technology in the target population is high—at the stage of "late majority"—but the application needs a continuous high-speed broadband connection to function. Unfortunately, due to financial reasons and overall infrastructure maturity, most target patients use older 3G networks, limiting the ability to implement the program in this area until 4G/5G network adoption increases or requiring program administrators to provide additional devices to ensure adequate broadband connection.

It is easy to miss differences in technology adoption between specific communities (Mars, 2013; Nwabueze et al., 2009), which can often lead to a widening of technology-driven disparities (Ortega et al., 2020). Often the differences in adoption of technology components may not be as evident as in the example above. A mandatory checklist should be adopted to ask "how" questions at every step in your technology workflow and assess whether the involved element's maturity can potentially influence the program's success.

For example, suppose that patients in the target population do not have timely access to a dermatologist. A new system can leverage machine learning to automatically triage all incoming images and facilitate the scheduling of appointments for at-risk patients. This system is potentially beneficial, but to ensure that the target population can effectively use the designed telemedicine program, a detailed step-by-step clinical workflow is developed to assess the adoption stage of every technology component used in the program. The analysis demonstrates that despite the high rate of adoption of smartphones and good penetration of high-speed data plans, the adoption of smartphones with high-resolution cameras is still low (early majority). In this target population, most users are extremely cost sensitive and use older or less expensive devices that will not provide the high-quality images required for successful image analysis. This low adoption of smartphones with high-resolution cameras can undoubtedly impact the program's success.

So far we have only discussed technological maturity from the patient's perspective, but the clinical environment can play an equally important role in a program's

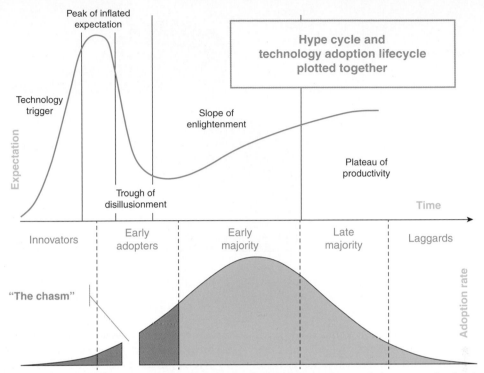

Fig. 8.5 Connection between the Gartner Cycle and Diffusion of Innovation graph, as a proxy for the size of the addressable market and readiness for technology adoption.

success (Marcin et al., 2016). Clinical environments follow similar maturity steps during their digital transformation journeys, and the availability of technology at a particular clinical site does not always reflect the site's ability to expand it or support additional clinical use cases. A hospital or a clinic may be in a different maturity stage, and any component of hospital digital infrastructure—such as clinical data warehouse, electronic medical record (EMR) adoption, video visits technology availability, and remote patient monitoring—can all influence the ability to create a successful telemedicine program.

Sometimes patients and clinical practices may be in different stages of technology adoption. The influence of external systems can shape patients' expectations related to clinical services. This factor often takes the form of "If I can do X, I should also be able to do Y." Unfortunately, healthcare institutions have historically paid less attention to the provision of a digital experience than retail, banking, or other consumer services. Disconnected technology adoption curves can explain this gap between patients' expectations and the available services between patients and healthcare institutions. Fig. 8.6 demonstrates this gap, when more progressive technology customers are ready for the next phase of technology innovation by clinical

providers, but healthcare institutions have not yet reached this digital transformation stage. On the flip side, this "adoption gap" is also a zone of innovation and opportunities, because the unsatisfied demand may be addressed by new technology entrants who may affect the status quo of traditional care delivery methods.

HOW TO THINK ABOUT TECHNOLOGY

Fig. 8.1 introduced a simple diagram reflecting the clinical encounter between a patient and a clinician via telemedicine. It is easy to focus only on the encounter's technology, but that would be a mistake. Technology not only connects a patient and a clinician; it connects the patient's environment with the clinician's environment. The selected technology should support both environments and provide a robust communication medium for all elements of a clinical encounter. When the environmental impact is neglected, "unforeseen" technical issues can lead to the low adoption of a telemedicine program or a dangerous loss in the quality of delivered care (LeRouge & Garfield, 2013).

It is helpful to develop a strategic approach to technology evaluation (Fig. 8.7). Starting with a technology evaluation in Phase I, telemedicine program administrators

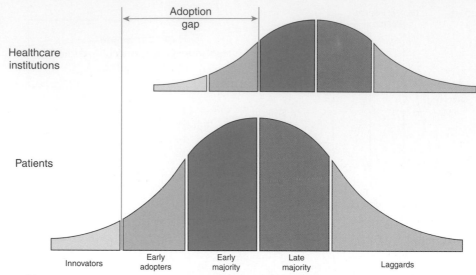

Fig. 8.6 Disconnect between adoption cycles between patients and clinical entities, which creates opportunities for disruptive innovation.

should ensure that the program meets target users' needs and adequately functions in the target environment. Next, in Phase II, evaluate whether the target technology is (or can be) used by the target population and if any efficacy signals can be attributed to the technology use. Lastly, in Phase III, evidence should be evaluated to confirm that the technology works not only in synthetic environments or preselected populations but also in the real world.

It is common to think about technology as a single element connecting participants during a clinical encounter, but that is a common misconception. Every telemedicine encounter is powered by a platform (a combination of technologies) that unifies multiple interconnected systems.

Every system involved in telemedicine visits should be independently evaluated to identify which technical elements could either be misaligned with one of the target environments or potentially cause technical issues. Unfortunately, it is often impossible to plan for all potential scenarios and address all future technology-related problems. Still, the presence of multiple points of failure highlights the need to understand the targeted user group and have a clear support plan for all issues encountered during the telemedicine visit (Bali, 2018).

EIGHT STEPS TO DEVELOP A TELEMEDICINE PROGRAM PLAN

With a variety of deployed technologies and target populations, telemedicine program implementation plans can vary significantly, but despite all the differences in the specific technology deployment, the general approach to telemedicine program development remains consistent.

Before initiating technology selection, the program leader should clearly understand the program goal and all the internal and external factors that may affect a program's success. It is recommended to approach this evaluation systematically and follow the recommended assessment steps.

As a first step, describe the problem the telemedicine program is trying to solve. Focused problem description can narrow the scope and define program boundaries. Next, users should be assessed, evaluated, and described. At this step, the program leader should try to understand the users involved in the telemedicine program. Instead of thinking about every unique user, it may be easier to create an archetype of a typical user. In its simplest form, an archetype is a way to describe your average user. Every program should have at least two user archetypes, one for a typical patient and one for a clinician; however, most programs would benefit from a more granular approach to the description of users.

After describing the users, the program leader should describe the environment and related cultural and technology variables at both origination and clinical sites. This description can help to understand better what can and cannot work for a particular environment. Often the easiest way to start is to describe a specific environment for the selected archetypes. Program leaders should specifically focus on variables that may limit the program's success, such as remote geographic location, poor connectivity, cultural barriers, low literacy, or low technology adoption.

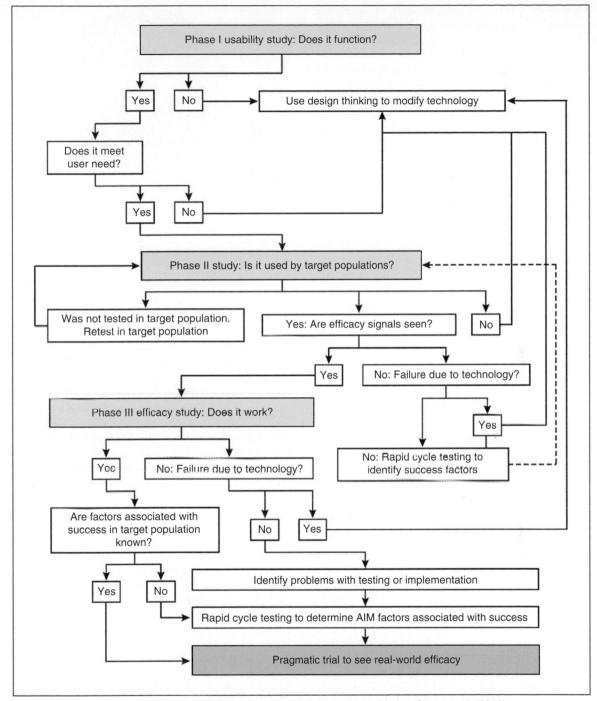

Fig. 8.7 Decision algorithm for digital health intervention validation. Sheon et al. (2018).

When both actors and environments are described, this information can be combined in a unified workflow diagram that depicts the process of telemedicine visit request and initiation, clinical information retrieval, clinical decision-making, prescription handling, and post-visit information communication. At this step, the goal is to understand the process in detail and ensure that all operational gaps are addressed. Your workflow can depict the user journey from both the patient and clinician sides. If necessary, additional actors can be added to step two to ensure that all the roles described in these steps have appropriate actors. It is cheaper to learn about potential barriers at the workflow design stage rather than after technology has been paid for and the program implemented. It is also helpful to draw a process for a technical support request or alternative communication options.

With a completed workflow diagram and a described set of actors, it is time to review the available tools and technical expertise. Not all new projects require new technology. Ideally, technology should be scaled across multiple use cases, simplifying long-term maintenance and the total cost of technology ownership. An additional benefit of widely implemented technology is the ability to develop internal expertise. Strong internal expertise, even in the absence of a full software development team, allows companies to architect and implement telemedicine projects better. Do not focus the search for expertise on "telemedicine champions" or technology innovators; it is more important to involve people who can ask the right questions, have broad clinical or technical expertise, and can bring an independent perspective to avoid the dreaded "group thinking."

By step six, the program leader should clearly understand the existing technology and technology gaps. The gap can be as big as a completely missing telemedicine platform or as small as a missing data analytics component for the remote patient monitoring program. The focus should not be on the perceived complexity of a missing technology element. Instead, it is critical to understand clearly what actions you want the system to perform and what results you expect to get. Using the information about currently available technology and any technology gap, the program leader can define the project's technological needs. Understanding the program needs allows a targeted search to be conducted for a technology solution. As we will discuss in the next step, an abundance of technology and vendors ready to solve any problem can easily create scope creep for the project. When this happens, the program team unintentionally loses focus and switches from solving a specific problem to planning the implementation of a particular, most often vendor-specific, technology. Telemedicine program leaders should never forget that technology should solve an existing problem, not create a new one.

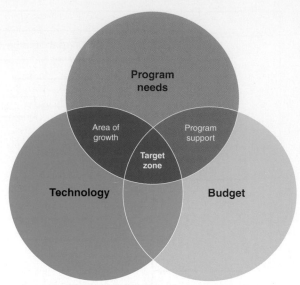

Fig. 8.8 Telehealth Technology Implementation targets.

After understanding program goals and technology needs, finally, technology and vendor can be selected. Value should guide the selection process, and can only be generated when the technology both is affordable and addresses the program's needs. Fig. 8.8 demonstrates the "target zone," an intersection of the program needs with available technologies that can be purchased within the budget constraints. Program leaders should focus on selecting technologies from the target zone and avoid spending time on others that are not affordable or not directly connected to the project goals. "Area of growth" represents tools and technologies for future considerations—the ones that may benefit the healthcare institution, but for financial or administrative reasons cannot be included in the scope of the current program.

Telemedicine program success depends not only on the deployment of a mature technology supported by both clinical environments but also on the leaders' ability to prepare the target users and their environments and provide long-term support. As the last step, the telemedicine leader should develop an implementation and support plan for the program. This plan should include a technology implementation plan, targeted educational activities, technology, clinical workflow validation, and a long-term support plan. A detailed discussion of project management activities related to the project implementation is out of scope for this chapter. Lastly, the role of training should not be underestimated, and targeted efforts should be made to ensure that clinicians are comfortable with their new technology-enabled clinical environments and can understand the basic troubleshooting steps.

In the next few sections, we will dive deeper into some of those steps and discuss other important components of a successful telemedicine program design and deployment.

Solve the Right Problem

As discussed earlier, while planning for any technology-enabled service, it is crucial to understand both users and the operational environment. Technology-first approaches rarely succeed, and telemedicine program leaders should ensure that the technology solves a problem rather than creating one.

Understand Your Problem

With the growing acceptance of telemedicine technologies among clinicians, administrators, and payers, it is easy to start with a "solution." Clinical leaders may see case studies in the literature and request to "enable video visits" or add "remote patient monitoring." Unfortunately, these kinds of initiatives rarely succeed. No matter how "easy" an initial problem appears, program leaders should always invest time to understand the problem in detail. Telemedicine-related technology is always just a component of a bigger puzzle, and every telemedicine program requires proper clinical workflow integrations and IT support.

For example, suppose you have been asked to enable remote patient monitoring for patients with congestive heart failure. Clinical service is looking for "just a few devices" to give at-risk patients the means to monitor their clinical symptoms and weight at home. The clinical sponsor believes these data can help them to find at-risk patients earlier and avoid hospital admissions.

In this scenario it would be easy to fall into the "simplicity" trap and provide monitoring devices without proper clinical workflows and technology integration. Unfortunately, this approach is unlikely to solve the problem. One of the essential pieces of information in this vignette is the program's desired outcome. The clinical champion wants to "decrease admissions," but the technology problem is not well defined. It is safe to assume a data gap between the patient and clinician, but what kind of data—and, most importantly, what specific data insights can prevent a hospital admission—is not yet clear.

Lastly, at this point, no information about the patients and their environments is available. We have seen that technology selection should be supported by the target environments and accepted by the target users. As discussed in the previous section, program leaders should go through the program design steps and fill the information gaps. When a completed workflow is designed, user archetypes can be used to evaluate your proposed solution from your target customer's viewpoint. This approach is especially helpful for launching a new program in an area with limited adoption of the selected technology.

For example, imagine you are leading a project focused on addressing limited clinical access in a remote village in Africa. You are considering using the telemedicine terminal to establish a face-to-face video chat with a remote clinician. Unfortunately, during the archetype creation, you realized your community has had little exposure to the technology before and "does not believe doctors from the screen."

The example above may be extreme, but it vividly illustrates a crucial point: both patients and clinical staff should trust the technology. In the example above, patients are not familiar with telemedicine clinical practice and do not believe that receiving care via a telemedicine channel is on a par with a traditional face-to-face visit. This disconnect highlights the importance of ensuring that the target environment not only supports the proposed solution from a technology perspective but accepts it from the clinical one.

How to Align Technology With the Local Environment

It is critical to align the telemedicine program's goals with the organization's mission, vision, and goals. As part of the strategic planning, the following aspects should be addressed:

- **Clinical strategy alignment.** Can a new telemedicine program provide safe and high-quality care for all participants irrespective of their technological expertise? Does the new system improve clinical outcomes? Does it improve access to care?
- **Financial strategy alignment.** Most telemedicine programs do not demonstrate a positive return on investment (ROI) within the first few years of operation. This financial implication should not be a barrier to adoption of the program if the long-term program benefits align with a strategic vision. Financial alignment can also help keep the program costs low because, especially for programs with limited technical expertise, an abundance of technical options can lead to overspending on technology. Notice that in Fig. 8.8, the "target zone" is significantly smaller than the "technology playground"—an area where purchased technology does not serve the immediate needs of a telemedicine program but is used more as a technology-focused experiment.
- **Technology strategy alignment.** Does the new telemedicine program integrate well with the current system? Can the same platform be expanded to multiple clinical service lines to create similar programs on the same technological base? Most clinical specialties and subspecialties have several vendors that provide a "tailored" solution to address the perceived uniqueness of clinical program

needs. Sometimes buying these targeted systems may be a good approach, but it can often lead to unnecessary technological fragmentation and growth in support costs. "Perceived uniqueness" is created by vendors as a marketing differentiation tool and can be addressed by bringing specific program needs to a common technology differentiator based on the clinical workflow. Leaders should select tools that provide enough customization flexibility to support future optimization requests to address programs' unique requirements.

How to Assess Your Technology Need

After developing a detailed understanding of the problem and the environmental factors that may influence implementation on both sides of clinical care (patient and clinician), it is time to explore technological solutions that can help to solve the problem. In most clinical settings, EMRs are at the center of clinical activities, and all technology assessments should start with a deep dive into current EMR capabilities.

Most modern EMRs support extensibility via proprietary integration technologies or modern integration frameworks (context-aware links, "SMART on FHIR" applications). Supported extensibility simplifies the integration of third-party applications and helps to provide users with a seamless clinical workflow.

When developing new technology-enabled services, organizations may encounter a classic "build versus buy" question. Unfortunately, there is no easy answer to this question, but an organization should carefully assess all available third-party options and internal technological expertise before considering self-developing a product (Lokken et al., 2020; Vega et al., 2013). Usually, the final decision depends on the answers to the following core questions:

1. What are the limitations of the solutions that are available on the market? How will those limitations impact the telemedicine program? Can clinical workflows be modified to suit the available technology solutions better?
2. What kind of integration is required from the application? Will the custom-built applications have access to all the required data, and what kind of additional integration layers will be required?
3. Does the organization have in-house access to the required talent? If not, can it attract and retain the talent required to develop and maintain the application?
4. What is the maintenance model? How dynamic is the implemented EMR system, and how much additional development effort will be required to keep the developed system operational?
5. What is the total cost of the project? (Include all the costs related to in-house development and maintenance.

Development rarely stops with a go-live—do not forget about the "area of growth" from Fig. 8.8—and system optimization beyond regular maintenance is a key component of successful projects.)

In complicated, multispecialty clinical settings, in-house development beyond clinical research or innovation is rarely the most cost-effective option. A large organization can often find a way to form a codevelopment partnership with a technology company to customize a current product or even develop a new one suitable for their specific clinical needs.

THE DOS AND DON'TS OF A PILOT PROGRAM

All telemedicine programs need a pilot. The pilot helps users achieve hands-on learning and allows technology innovators to validate their assumptions (Arnold et al., 2009; Thabane et al., 2010). Technology innovators learn by pilots (Arain et al., 2010). However, there is a big problem: pilots are hard to plan and even harder to execute (Moore et al., 2011). Most healthcare institutions use "pilot" as a generic term for anything related to the limited implementation of a new workflow. The caveat is that a pilot lacking a hypothesis, defined success metrics, key performance indicators, and the perspective scale plan is just a waste of time (Shanyinde et al., 2011). A pilot is a learning exercise (Sheon et al., 2018). It is a core experimental element in a "fail fast" strategy, and it should be treated that way. A well-designed pilot can help a team to learn fast and discover potential problems with technology vendors, clinical workflow, or any other aspects of their telemedicine program early.

What Is a Pilot?

Pilot testing is a learning tool based on the limited deployment of a technology or program to a selected group of early users (Thabane et al., 2010). The limited nature of the engagement allows program administrators to learn from real interaction on a limited scale. During the pilot, one or several components of the program are tested; this could include technology or clinical workflows and integrations.

Qualities of a Good Pilot

A good pilot and good research have one thing in common: a hypothesis (Arain et al., 2010; Van Teijlingen & Hundley, 2002). A hypothesis is anything that can be reliably proved or disproved during the testing period. For example, it could be a technology-focused hypothesis that "technology X can reliably work in the environment Y," an operational-focused one that "program X can provide virtual cardiac rehab services asynchronously," or even a clinical workflow–focused one that "wearable sensor X can reliably collect data element Y for clinical decision-making." Most importantly, the hypothesis should be specific and testable. Broad "pseudo-pilots" lacking hypotheses and timelines are often just poor deployment programs that waste time and resources and do not provide learning or clinical benefits.

How to Design a Pilot

The pilot is a focused learning exercise. When planning for the pilot:
1. Define the hypothesis and set a clear learning goal.
2. Constrain the pilot in time and deployment scale (focus on a specific group of users or a particular problem).
3. Design an effective data collection and feedback loop.

The Danger of No-Learning Pilots

As mentioned before, a pilot is a learning exercise (Moore et al., 2011). A pilot is also a chance to test training materials and support mechanisms or validate new technology. Poorly deployed programs without learning components are not pilots. The term "pilot" has been commonly overused and assigned to poorly planned programs with minimal deployment support, or programs with no scale potential. Piloting just for a pilot's sake generates waste and needlessly burns out users involved in a project.

Death by Pilot

Poorly designed and planned pilots are harmful not only to healthcare institutions but also to the technology or services companies powering the program (Van Teijlingen & Hundley, 2001). Many digital health innovators are afraid of the dreaded "death by pilot" that happens when a young, innovative company with promising technology runs out of resources before generating any value. It is often a result of the notoriously long sell cycle in the healthcare industry; however, a more common reason is a poorly planned pilot with no immediate problem to solve, poorly defined goals and performance indicators, and no clear pathway for scaling a program.

Learning From Your Pilot

It is crucial to define optimal learning mechanisms and corresponding data collection streams during the pilot design stage. Data collection should be at the center of the pilot efforts. Users should have an easy workflow that allows them to provide feedback in addition to regular structured feedback sessions. All collected information should be analyzed and combined in the form of actionable "lessons learned" recommendations. Ideally, the pilot results should be widely communicated across the organization to stimulate collective learning and avoid repeating discovered problems. Program workflow and technology assumptions should be modified based on the pilot's results. If the

system performed well according to previously defined key performance indicators (KPIs) and project goals, the project can proceed to the next scaling step; if not, the program should be modified and prepared for another pilot.

COST OF SYSTEM OWNERSHIP

Earlier we discussed the importance of aligning user needs and technology options with the budget. Program sustainability depends on its ability to generate a sustainable ROI. For programs where ROI is hard to calculate, generated clinical value or volume-related clinical metrics can be implemented, but in any scenario, programs require a financial contribution to support technology and personnel-related costs. It is essential to calculate costs for a pilot period and a future deployment at scale. Vendors may often offer unrealistically attractive terms for a pilot deployment, so calculating the total cost of ownership helps program managers to look past the pilot stage. While estimating the total cost of ownership, the following costs should be considered:

- Infrastructure costs: Updating on-premise servers or purchasing cloud infrastructure will have associated costs. How easily can the infrastructure be scaled up if the program grows?
- Software license cost: How does the vendor charge for a license? Is it based on an enterprise license or charged per user per month? If the program starts small, ensure that scaling up the program is financially sustainable. What is the software update structure, and how does the vendor charge for a new version?
- Implementation costs: Pilot projects are often conducted with minimal implementation. Though it carries less financial risk, be aware that a less integrated workflow can often lead to poor user experience and pilot failure.
- Security costs: Are any additional security tools or certifications required? Could this program introduce a new vulnerability vector? Does this new deployment require the system to expand the audit program? Does it increase overall security risks? If yes, can those new risks negatively affect cyberinsurance risk premiums?
- Training and support costs: How much additional support does the program require to deploy the selected technology successfully? What proportion of the support can be provided by internal resources, and what needs a separate support agreement from a vendor? Is training included in the platform cost? What support is provided as part of a license during software updates, and what should be purchased separately? What training materials are available?

IMPLEMENTATION PLANNING

Even a good telemedicine program can fail due to poor implementation (Grigsby et al., 2007; Yellowlees, 2005). A comprehensive discussion of a telemedicine program go-live requires a dedicated chapter, but we will briefly highlight some technology-related points telemedicine program leaders should keep in mind.

"People, processes, and technology" is a methodology that highlights the balance between the project's critical elements (Humphrey, 1988; Sharma, 2005). Commonly referred to as a "golden triangle," the combination of people, process, and technology requires coordination of efforts on every side of the triangle to achieve success. This point is critical to remember when planning for the implementation of a new telemedicine program. Stellar technology alone cannot make the program successful without the people (inadequate training, poor customer support, etc.) or process (fragmented integration, inconsistent clinical workflow) components. Even in a technology-focused role, a program leader should ensure that all elements of this "golden triangle" are appropriately addressed and aligned.

PROGRAM GOVERNANCE

An effective governance structure is an essential component of program management and can define program success. Traditionally, the following roles are critical for program design and implementation:

- Clinical champion: The program needs a clinical leader with deep expertise in the target clinical domain and a good understanding of the selected technology. The clinical champion's primary goal is to design and validate technology-enabled workflows and serve as a local leader during implementation. Program leaders should carefully select clinical champions and ensure the selected individuals are willing to support the project at scale and have the necessary bandwidth to do it.
- Executive sponsor: A successful program needs significant support from executive leadership. This role is especially important for programs with a negative ROI, or very innovative technologies or workflows.
- Telehealth program manager: Program administration requires the tracking of program performance and developing and maintaining the required documentation.
- Telehealth trainer: Peer-to-peer training is essential, and having a dedicated trainer familiar with the selected technology and designed clinical workflow can be the difference between a program's success and failure.

TECHNICAL SUPPORT AND BASIC TROUBLESHOOTING

Every telemedicine program encounters a technology-related service interruption (Craig & Patterson, 2005; Elliott & Yopes, 2019). Service failure could result from an individual operator error (e.g., a patient who cannot correctly install a required mobile application or enable video camera access in the browser) or a system error, where one or multiple technical factors make the system unusable (e.g., internet service failure or failure of a telemedicine platform cloud infrastructure) (Broens et al., 2007). The difference between a well-organized telemedicine program and a poorly planned one is the robustness of the available technical support and preparedness of the key personnel to deal with technical problems (Field, 1996; Yellowlees, 2005). Patient safety should remain the key focus of all clinical encounters, and alternative communication methods should be established to provide clinical care in case of telemedicine platform malfunction. The variety of consumer devices and the variability of potential technical configurations make technology-specific troubleshooting challenging for nontechnical users. All telemedicine programs should have dedicated support lines to provide technical guidance for both patients and clinicians. Sometimes it may be cost-effective to outsource technical support directly to telemedicine platform vendors with deep expertise in handling technology-related problems and experience in running a support line (Jennett et al., 2003).

When basic video troubleshooting is required, clinicians should follow the following troubleshooting steps:

1. Ensure that the clinical device is running correctly and not in the process of a system upgrade. When appropriate, attempt to restart the device.
2. Verify an internet connection. Some devices may be set up to only work on specific networks; in this case, verify that the device is connected to an appropriate network.
3. Check internet speed. Poor internet speed is the most common reason for failure or low quality of video visits.
4. If the application runs in a browser, ensure that browser windows have access to audio and video devices. Usually, only one application can have access to audio and video streams. Check whether other browser tabs or applications are currently using your devices.

These steps can also be generalized to the following: users should ensure that the device is running correctly, then ensure an internet connection is available and meets the minimum connection requirement, then check that the telemedicine application is launched and has all the necessary devices access rights (video camera, microphone, speakers, or other connected devices). If necessary, similar troubleshooting steps should be repeated on both sides of the telemedicine connection.

Troubleshooting beyond basic steps is challenging and should be performed by certified technicians who understand both the technology and the telemedicine platform. Fortunately, most technical problems are self-limited and can be addressed by following the directions provided to users during implementation training.

SECURITY AND THE HEALTH INSURANCE PORTABILITY AND ACCOUNTABILITY ACT

In the United States, the Health Insurance Portability and Accountability Act (HIPAA) defines the set of healthcare industry-wide standards for the handling of protected health information. HIPAA was passed in 1996, but to incorporate the growing requirements, multiple updates were introduced over the years: HIPAA Privacy Rule in 2003, HIPAA Security Rule in 2005, and most recently, the Health Information Technology for Economic and Clinical Health (HITEC) act in 2013 (Annas, 2003; Atchinson & Fox, 1997; Gostin et al., 2009).

Under HIPAA, protected health information is defined as individually identifiable information related to an individual's health status or the delivered care created, collected, or transmitted by a HIPAA-covered entity. Protected health information is defined as health information that includes discoverable identifiers (e.g., name, social security number, phone number; for the full list of HIPAA identifiers, please refer to Appendix 1). If none of those identifiers are present, the information is considered deidentified protected health information.

However, HIPAA rules only apply to "covered entities" and their "business associates," so small digital health applications may not need HIPAA compliance, which can introduce privacy risks for healthcare organizations and patients. Under HIPAA, only health plans, healthcare clearinghouses, and most healthcare providers are considered covered entities. Vendors and software development partners are considered business associates of the covered entity, and this kind of arrangement requires a written agreement between the service provider and the covered entity (Lawson et al., 2003).

Keep in mind that HIPAA regulates all protected health information that is held or transmitted by a covered entity or its business associate and not specific to any particular mode of information transfer. This means that HIPAA applies to any form of information transfer, whether electronic, paper, or even oral.

Privacy

HIPAA compliance does not guarantee compliance with other privacy requirements. This diversity of requirements is especially important to understand when engaging a new technology vendor with limited experience in your region. As a program leader, it is your responsibility to ensure that the selected technology complies with local requirements and has the necessary certification (Luxton et al., 2012).

Data privacy is a dynamic field, and your institution should have guidelines and recommendations addressing the recommended data handling standards. These recommendations should be used to guide the discussions about data sharing (private and anonymous), data ownership, and data/insight reselling (Gostin et al., 2009; Hall & McGraw, 2014).

SUMMARY

Technology plays a critical role in every telemedicine program. Telemedicine programs are powered by technology; however, it is essential to understand that a program is more than just the sum of all related tools. Leaders responsible for designing telemedicine programs should pay attention to the environment where the selected technology will be deployed and the adoption cycle stage. A disconnect between patients' and healthcare institutions' adoption cycles can make program design particularly challenging. Growing technological demands may push the requirements outside current technical capabilities. Discovered technology gaps should be not only addressed on the individual program level but incorporated into a global digital transformation plan.

Every new technology should be internally evaluated and an assessment made of whether it needs to be validated, piloted, or scaled. If the technology was never used in clinical settings before, it should be validated before a pilot or deployment into a clinical program. A pilot is a learning tool to test program assumptions and evaluate a program on a limited scale. Every pilot should have a clear goal, a dedicated pilot team, and a set of KPIs.

"Build versus buy" is not an easy decision and should be driven by internal resource availability and the total cost of ownership. Internally built platforms can be more expensive in the long run due to growing support costs.

During the implementation stage, particular attention should be paid to training and customer support. The "train the trainer" model helps mobilize internal resources and increase internal product expertise.

When creating a technology architecture for a telemedicine program, the program leader should always focus on the customers. The goal is to understand the problem and any additional requirements created by the target environment. "Fail fast" does not mean focusing on failure; it means bringing a product to customers for feedback as soon as possible. When possible, design and prototype on paper.

When designing a telemedicine program, do not focus on the technology. Remember that technology is just an intermediate layer that can bring clinical environments together to make care more affordable, accessible, and safe.

KEY POINTS

- Technology powers telemedicine programs but should not define them.
- Clear understanding of the telemedicine program goal is required to define the scope.
- A combination of clinical and technical expertise is essential for the long-term program success
- Solve the right problem – technology by itself is rarely an answer. Focus on the clinical or operational needs
- Properly designed and implemented telemedicine technology should not disturb the clinical practice but instead augment it by bringing care closer to patients
- The patient should be in the center of innovation, and access barriers should be assessed during every step of the program design to avoid the digital divide

- The Technology Adoption gap by healthcare institutions creates an opportunity for innovation-driven by patients' demand
- To avoid "death by pilots," conduct well-defined pilots with clear learning objectives
- Every program should have documented governance structure with periodic reviews of key performance indicators. Program iteration is critical for success.
- Good training coupled with ongoing support can be the difference between the program success and failure
- Design the system to protect the privacy and security of your patients. Always ensure that every product you use and every vendor you work with complies with the security and privacy requirements.

⑦ CRITICAL THINKING EXERCISES

- You are tasked to design a clinical program to provide prenatal monitoring of high-risk pregnancies in rural Mexico. Your hospital is located in New York, and care will be provided by a combination of medical residents and advance practice providers. The project goal is to detect at-risk patients early, counseling and clinical care
  - What questions would you like to ask the local program administrators to start program planning?
  - What barriers to adoption do you foresee, and what can you do to address it?
  - What technological approaches do you think will work, and which ones will not? Why?

- Your local innovation center wants to implement a new, artificial intelligence-powered platform that can provide proactive monitoring of at-risk patients with congestive heart failure. At this point, the project does not have buy-in from the local clinicians, and no clinical champions have been identified.
  - How will you approach the implementation of this project?
  - What key performance indicators can you recommend for the pilot?
  - What barriers to the adoption do you foresee, and what can you do to address them?

REVIEW QUESTIONS

1. The ambulatory surgical center is looking to evaluate patients remotely before the procedure. They are looking for an easy-to-use technology solution that can provide real-time video visits, but do not have a dedicated budget. What should you do next?
   a. Meet with the group to understand the problem, but because they have no budget, recommend using free video technology like Skype or Facetime.

   b. Meet with the group, understand the problem, and request a budget because it is required for the implementation of enterprise-level video communication technology.
   c. Meet with the group, understand the problem, and start discussing the patients covered by the service live.
   d. Request additional information from the service line. Explain that potential financial impact needs

to be calculated before you can start any technical discussion.

2. Why would you conduct a pilot?
   a. To evaluate the selected vendor and related technology.
   b. To conduct an experiment and validate a hypothesis.
   c. To deploy your program slowly.
   d. To save money on the full deployment.
3. You are providing telemedicine coverage for a virtual urgent care clinic. Your telemedicine application is running in the browser, and up to this point, you have successfully provided five telemedicine visits. On your sixth visit, you can hear your patient, but the video is not available. What should you do next?
   a. Ask the patient to call again.
   b. Decline the consult because the video is not available.
   c. Ask if any other video conferencing software is running in the background and may be using the camera.
   d. Ask about the speed of the patient's internet connection.

APPENDIX 1 HIPAA IDENTIFIERS

1. Names (full or last name and initial).
2. All geographical identifiers smaller than a state, except for the initial three digits of a zip code if, according to the current publicly available data from the US Bureau of the Census, the geographic unit formed by combining all zip codes with the same three initial digits contains more than 20,000 people; the initial three digits of a zip code for all such geographic units containing 20,000 or fewer people is changed to 000.
3. Dates (other than year) directly related to an individual.
4. Phone numbers.
5. Fax numbers.
6. Email addresses.
7. Social Security numbers.
8. Medical record numbers.
9. Health insurance beneficiary numbers.
10. Account numbers.
11. Certificate/license numbers.
12. Vehicle identifiers (including serial numbers and license plate numbers).
13. Device identifiers and serial numbers.
14. Web Uniform Resource Locators (URLs).
15. IP address numbers.
16. Biometric identifiers, including finger, retinal, and voice prints.
17. Full face photographic images and any comparable images.
18. Any other unique identifying number, characteristic, or code except the unique code assigned by the investigator to code the data.

REFERENCES

AAMC. (2021). *Telehealth competencies across the learning continuum. AAMC New and Emerging Areas in Medicine Series.* Washington, DC: AAMC.

Annas, G. J. (2003). HIPAA regulations – a new era of medical-record privacy? *New England Journal of Medicine, 348*(15), 1486–1490. https://doi.org/10.1056/NEJMlim035027

Arain, M., Campbell, M. J., Cooper, C. L., et al. (2010). What is a pilot or feasibility study? A review of current practice and editorial policy. *BMC Medical Research Methodology, 10*, 67. https://doi.org/10.1186/1471-2288-10-67

Arnold, D. M., Burns, K. E. A., Adhikari, N. K. J., et al. (2009). The design and interpretation of pilot trials in clinical research in critical care. *Critical Care Medicine, 37*(Suppl. 1), S69–S74. https://doi.org/10.1097/CCM.0b013e3181920e33

Atchinson, B. K., & Fox, D. M. (1997). From the field: The politics of the health insurance portability and accountability act. *Health Affairs, 16*(3), 146–150. https://doi.org/10.1377/hlthaff.16.3.146

Aziz, A., Zork, N., Aubey, J. J., et al. (2020). Telehealth for high-risk pregnancies in the setting of the COVID-19 pandemic. *American Journal of Perinatology, 37*(8), 800–808. https://doi.org/10.1055/s-0040-1712121

Bali, S. (2018). Barriers to development of telemedicine in developing countries. *Telehealth IntechOpen.*

Barao, S. M. (1992). Behavioral aspects of technology adoption: the role of on-farm demonstration. *Journal of Extension, 30*(2), 13–15.

Bashshur, R. L. (1995). On the definition and evaluation of telemedicine. *Telemedicine Journal, 1*(1), 19–30. https://doi.org/10.1089/tmj.1.1995.1.19.

Bashshur, R. L., Shannon, G. W., Smith, B. R., et al. (2014). The empirical foundations of telemedicine interventions for chronic disease management. *Telemedicine Journal and e-Health, 20*(9), 769–800. https://doi.org/10.1089/tmj.2014.9981.

Broens, T. H. F., Huis in't Veld, R. M. H. A., Vollenbroek-Hutten, M. M. R., et al. (2007). Determinants of successful telemedicine implementations: A literature study. *Journal of Telemedicine and Telecare, 13*(6), 303–309. https://doi.org/10.1258/135763307781644951

Canfield, C., & Galvin, S. (2018). Bedside nurse acceptance of intensive care unit telemedicine presence. *Critical Care Nurse, 38*(6), e1–e4. https://doi.org/10.4037/ccn2018926

Celler, B. G., Lovell, N. H., & Basilakis, J. (2003). Using information technology to improve the management of chronic disease. *Medical Journal of Australia*, *179*(5), 242–246. https://doi.org/10.5694/j.1326-5377.2003.tb05529.x

Chaudoir, S. R., Dugan, A. G., & Barr, C. H. I. (2013). Measuring factors affecting implementation of health innovations: A systematic review of structural, organizational, provider, patient, and innovation level measures. *Implementation Science*, *8*, 22. https://doi.org/10.1186/1748-5908-8-22

Connolly, S. L., Stolzmann, K. L., Heyworth, L., et al. (2021). Rapid increase in telemental health within the Department of Veterans Affairs during the COVID-19 pandemic. *Telemedicine Journal and e-Health*, *27*(4), 454–458. https://doi.org/10.1089/tmj.2020.0233.

Craig, J., & Patterson, V. (2005). Introduction to the practice of telemedicine. *Journal of Telemedicine and Telecare*, *11*(1), 3–9. https://doi.org/10.1177/1357633X0501100102

Cranen, K., Veld, R. H. I., Ijzerman, M., et al. (2011). Change of patients' perceptions of telemedicine after brief use. *Telemedicine Journal and e-Health*, *17*(7), 530–535. https://doi.org/10.1089/tmj.2010.0208.

Criner, G. J., Bourbeau, J., Diekemper, R. L., et al. (2015). Prevention of acute exacerbations of COPD: American College of Chest Physicians and Canadian Thoracic Society guideline. *Chest*, *147*(4), 894–942. https://doi.org/10.1378/chest.14-1676

Darkins, A., Ryan, P., Kobb, R., et al. (2008). Care coordination/home telehealth: The systematic implementation of health informatics, home telehealth, and disease management to support the care of veteran patients with chronic conditions. *Telemedicine Journal and e-Health*, *14*(10), 1118–1126. https://doi.org/10.1089/tmj.2008.0021.

de Bustos, E. M., Moulin, T., & Audebert, H. J. (2009). Barriers, legal issues, limitations and ongoing questions in telemedicine applied to stroke. *Cerebrovascular Diseases*, *27*(Suppl. 4), 36–39. https://doi.org/10.1159/000213057.

Dedehayir, O., & Steinert, M. (2016). The hype cycle model: A review and future directions. *Technological Forecasting and Social Change*, *108*(C), 28–41. https://econpapers.repec.org/RePEc:eee:tefoso:v:108:y:2016:i:c:p:28-41.

Duncan, N. B. (1995). Capturing flexibility of information technology infrastructure: A study of resource characteristics and their measure. *Journal of Management Information Systems*, *12*(2), 37–57. https://doi.org/10.1080/07421222.1995.11518080

Eedy, D. J., & Wootton, R. (2001). Teledermatology: A review. *British Journal of Dermatology*, *144*(4), 696–707. https://doi.org/10.1046/j.1365-2133.2001.04124.x

Elliott, T., & Yopes, M. C. (2019). Direct-to-consumer telemedicine. *Journal of Allergy and Clinical Immunology: In Practice*, *7*(8), 2546–2552. https://doi.org/10.1016/j.jaip.2019.06.027

Field, M. J. (1996). *Telemedicine: A guide to assessing telecommunications for health care*. Washington, DC: National Academy Press. https://doi.org/10.17226/5296.

Fogel, A., Khamisa, K., Afkham, A., et al. (2017). Ask the eConsultant: Improving access to haematology expertise using an asynchronous eConsult system. *Journal of Telemedicine and Telecare*, *23*(3), 421–427. https://doi.org/10.1177/1357633X16644095

Gostin, L. O., Levit, L. A., & Nass, S. J. (Eds.). (2009). *Beyond the HIPAA privacy rule: Enhancing privacy, improving health through research*. Washington, DC: National Academy Press.

Greenhalgh, T., Wherton, J., Shaw, S., et al. (2020). Video consultations for covid-19. *BMJ (Clinical Research Ed.)*, *368*, m998. https://doi.org/10.1136/bmj.m998

Grigsby, B., Brega, A. G., Bennett, R. E., et al. (2007). The slow pace of interactive video telemedicine adoption: The perspective of telemedicine program administrators on physician participation. *Telemedicine Journal and e-Health: The Official Journal of the American Telemedicine Association*, *13*(6), 645–656. https://doi.org/10.1089/tmj.2007.0090.

Grundy, B. L., Crawford, P., Jones, P. K., et al. (1977). Telemedicine in critical care: An experiment in health care delivery. *Journal of the American College of Emergency Physicians*, *6*(10), 439–444. https://doi.org/10.1016/s0361-1124(77)80239-6

Grundy, B. L., Jones, P. K., & Lovitt, A. (1982). Telemedicine in critical care: Problems in design, implementation, and assessment. *Critical Care Medicine*, *10*(7), 471–475. https://doi.org/10.1097/00003246-198207000-00014

Hailey, D., Roine, R., & Ohinmaa, A. (2002). Systematic review of evidence for the benefits of telemedicine. *Journal of Telemedicine and Telecare*, *8*(Suppl. 1), 1–30. https://doi.org/10.1258/1357633021937604

Hall, J. L., & McGraw, D. (2014). For telehealth to succeed, privacy and security risks must be identified and addressed. *Health Affairs (Project Hope)*, *33*(2), 216–221. https://doi.org/10.1377/hlthaff.2013.0997

Harst, L., Lantzsch, H., & Scheibe, M. (2019). Theories predicting end-user acceptance of telemedicine use: Systematic review. *Journal of Medical Internet Research*, *21*(5), e13117. https://doi.org/10.2196/13117

Holden, D., & Dew, E. (2008). Telemedicine in a rural gero-psychiatric inpatient unit: Comparison of perception/satisfaction to onsite psychiatric care. *Telemedicine Journal and e-Health*, *14*(4), 381–384. https://doi.org/10.1089/tmj.2007.0054.

Hollander, J. E., & Carr, B. G. (2020). Virtually perfect? Telemedicine for COVID-19. *New England Journal of Medicine*, *382*(18), 1679–1681. https://doi.org/10.1056/NEJMp2003539

Humphrey, W. S. (1988). Characterizing the software process: A maturity framework. *IEEE Software*, *5*(2), 73–79. https://doi.org/10.1109/52.2014

Jennett, P., Yeo, M., Pauls, M., et al. (2003). Organizational readiness for telemedicine: Implications for success and failure. *Journal of Telemedicine and Telecare*, *9*(Suppl. 2), S27–S30. https://doi.org/10.1258/135763303322596183

Jones, A., Hedges-Chou, J., Bates, J., et al. (2014). Home telehealth for chronic disease management: Selected findings of a narrative synthesis. *Telemedicine Journal and e-Health*, *20*(4), 346–380. https://doi.org/10.1089/tmj.2013.0249.

Karahanna, E., Straub, D. W., & Chervany, N. L. (1999). Information technology adoption across time: A cross-sectional comparison of pre-adoption and post-adoption beliefs. *Management Information Systems Quarterly*, *23*(2), 183–213. https://doi.org/10.2307/249751

Lawson, N. A., Orr, J. M., & Klar, D. S. (2003). The HIPAA privacy rule: An overview of compliance initiatives and requirements. *Definition of counsel*, *70*, 127.

Laxminarayan, S., & Istepanian, R. S. (2000). Unwired e-MED: The next generation of wireless and internet telemedicine systems. *IEEE Transactions on Information Technology in Biomedicine: A Publication of the IEEE Engineering in Medicine and Biology Society*, *4*(3), 189–193. https://doi.org/10.1109/titb.2000.5956074.

LeRouge, C., & Garfield, M. J. (2013). Crossing the telemedicine chasm: Have the U.S. Barriers to widespread adoption of telemedicine been significantly reduced? *International Journal of Environmental Research and Public Health*, *10*(12), 6472–6484. https://doi.org/10.3390/ijerph10126472

Liddy, C., Moroz, I., Mihan, A., et al. (2019). A systematic review of asynchronous, provider-to-provider, electronic consultation services to improve access to specialty care available worldwide. *Telemedicine Journal and e-Health*, *25*(3), 184–198. https://doi.org/10.1089/tmj.2018.0005.

Linden, A., & Fenn, J. (2003). *Understanding Gartner's hype cycles. Strategic Analysis Report Nº R-20-1971* (Vol. 88). Gartner, Inc, 1423.

Lokken, T. G., Blegen, R. N., Hoff, M. D., et al. (2020). Overview for implementation of telemedicine services in a large integrated multispecialty health care system. *Telemedicine Journal and e-Health*, *26*(4), 382–387. https://doi.org/10.1089/tmj.2019.0079.

Lovett, J. E., & Bashshur, R. L. (1979). Telemedicine in the USA: An overview. *Telecommunications Policy*, *3*(1), 3–14. https://doi.org/10.1016/0308-5961(79)90019-3

Luxton, D. D., Kayl, R. A., & Mishkind, M. C. (2012). mHealth data security: The need for HIPAA-compliant standardization. *Telemedicine Journal and e-Health*, *18*(4), 284–288. https://doi.org/10.1089/tmj.2011.0180.

Marcin, J. P., Shaikh, U., & Steinhorn, R. H. (2016). Addressing health disparities in rural communities using telehealth. *Pediatric Research*, *79*(1–2), 169–176. https://doi.org/10.1038/pr.2015.192

Mars, M. (2013). Telemedicine and advances in urban and rural healthcare delivery in Africa. *Progress in Cardiovascular Diseases*, *56*(3), 326–335. https://doi.org/10.1016/j.pcad.2013.10.006

Miller, E. A. (2003). The technical and interpersonal aspects of telemedicine: Effects on doctor–patient communication. *Journal of Telemedicine and Telecare*, *9*(1), 1–7. https://doi.org/10.1258/135763303321159611

Mohamed, S., & Rubino, G. (2002). A study of real-time packet video quality using random neural networks. *IEEE Transactions on Circuits and Systems for Video Technology*, *12*(12), 1071–1083. https://doi.org/10.1109/TCSVT.2002.806808

Moore, C. G., Carter, R. E., Nietert, P. J., et al. (2011). Recommendations for planning pilot studies in clinical and translational research. *Clinical and Translational Science*, *4*(5), 332–337. https://doi.org/10.1111/j.1752-8062.2011.00347.x

Najafi, B., Swerdlow, M., Murphy, G. A., et al. (2021). The promise and hurdles of telemedicine in diabetes foot care delivery. In *Telemedicine, telehealth and telepresence* (pp. 455–470). Cham, Switzerland: Springer Nature.

Newton, M. J. (2014). The promise of telemedicine. *Survey of Ophthalmology*, *59*(5), 559–567. https://doi.org/10.1016/j.survophthal.2014.02.003

Nittari, G., Khuman, R., Baldoni, S., et al. (2020). Telemedicine practice: Review of the current ethical and legal challenges. *Telemedicine Journal and e-Health*, *26*(12), 1427–1437. https://doi.org/10.1089/tmj.2019.0158.

Nwabueze, S., Meso, P., Mbarika, V., et al. (2009). The effects of culture of adoption of telemedicine in medically underserved communities. In *2009 42nd Hawaii International conference on system sciences*. https://doi.org/10.1109/HICSS.2009.430.

Ohannessian, R., Duong, T. A., & Odone, A. (2020). Global telemedicine implementation and integration within health systems to fight the COVID-19 pandemic: A call to action. *JMIR Public Health and Surveillance*, *6*(2), e18810. https://doi.org/10.2196/18810

O'Leary, D. E. (2008). Gartner's hype cycle and information system research issues. *International Journal of Accounting Information Systems*, *9*(4), 240–252.

Ortega, G., Rodriguez, J. A., Maurer, L. R., et al. (2020). Telemedicine, COVID-19, and disparities: Policy implications. *Health Policy and Technology*, *9*(3), 368–371. https://doi.org/10.1016/j.hlpt.2020.08.001

Perednia, D. A., & Allen, A. (1995). Telemedicine technology and clinical applications. *The Journal of the American Medical Association*, *273*(6), 483–488.

Perednia, D. A., & Brown, N. A. (1995). Teledermatology: One application of telemedicine. *Bulletin of the Medical Library Association*, *83*(1), 42–47.

Peters, C., Blohm, I., & Leimeister, J. M. (2015). Anatomy of successful business models for complex services: Insights from the telemedicine field. *Journal of Management Information Systems*, *32*(3), 75–104.

Pollard, S. E., & LePage, J. P. (2001). *Telepsychiatry in a rural inpatient setting Psychiatric Services (Washington, DC)*, *52*, 1659. https://doi.org/10.1176/appi.ps.52.12.1659-a.

Resneck, J. S. J., Abrouk, M., Steuer, M., et al. (2016). Choice, transparency, coordination, and quality among direct-to-consumer telemedicine websites and apps treating skin disease. *JAMA Dermatology*, *152*(7), 768–775. https://doi.org/10.1001/jamadermatol.2016.1774

Rogerts, E. M. (1995). Diffusion of innovations. Simon and Schruster, New York: Free Press.

Salisbury, C., Thomas, C., O'Cathain, A., et al. (2015). TElehealth in CHronic disease: Mixed-methods study to develop the TECH conceptual model for intervention design and evaluation. *BMJ Open*, *5*(2), e006448. https://doi.org/10.1136/bmjopen-2014-006448

Seufert, M., Egger, S., Slanina, M., et al. (2014). A survey on quality of experience of HTTP adaptive streaming. *IEEE Communications Surveys and Tutorials, 17*(1), 469–492.

Shanyinde, M., Pickering, R. M., & Weatherall, M. (2011). Questions asked and answered in pilot and feasibility randomized controlled trials. *BMC Medical Research Methodology, 11*, 117. https://doi.org/10.1186/1471-2288-11-117

Sharma, A. (2005). Collaborative product innovation: Integrating elements of CPI via PLM framework. *Computer-Aided Design, 37*(13), 1425–1434.

Sheon, A. R., Van Winkle, B., Solad, Y., et al. (2018). An algorithm for digital medicine testing: A NODE.health perspective intended to help emerging technology companies and healthcare systems navigate the trial and testing period prior to full-scale adoption. *Digital Biomarkers, 2*(3), 139–154. https://doi.org/10.1159/000494365

Sood, S., Mbarika, V., Jugoo, S., et al. (2007). What is telemedicine? A collection of 104 peer-reviewed perspectives and theoretical underpinnings. *Telemedicine Journal and e-Health, 13*(5), 573–590. https://doi.org/10.1089/tmj.2006.0073.

Stanberry, B. (2006). Legal and ethical aspects of telemedicine. *Journal of Telemedicine and Telecare, 12*(4), 166–175. https://doi.org/10.1258/135763306777488825

Straub, E. T. (2009). Understanding technology adoption: Theory and future directions for informal learning. *Review of Educational Research, 79*(2), 625–649.

Thabane, L., Ma, J., Chu, R., et al. (2010). A tutorial on pilot studies: The what, why and how. *BMC Medical Research Methodology, 10*, 1. https://doi.org/10.1186/1471-2288-10-1

Thomas, E. E., Haydon, H. M., Mehrotra, A., et al. (2020). Building on the momentum: Sustaining telehealth beyond COVID-19. *Journal of Telemedicine and Telecare*, 1357633X20960638. https://doi.org/10.1177/1357633X20960638.

Uscher-Pines, L., Mulcahy, A., Cowling, D., et al. (2016). Access and quality of care in direct-to-consumer telemedicine. *Telemedicine Journal and e-Health, 22*(4), 282–287. https://doi.org/10.1089/tmj.2015.0079.

Van Dyk, L. (2013). *The development of a telemedicine service maturity model.* [Doctoral dissertation] Stellenbosch University.

Van Lente, H., Spitters, C., & Peine, A. (2013). Comparing technological hype cycles: Towards a theory. *Technological Forecasting and Social Change, 80*(8), 1615–1628.

Van Teijlingen, E. R., & Hundley, V. (2001). The importance of conducting and reporting pilot studies: the example of the Scottish Births Survey. *Journal of advanced nursing, 34*(3), 289–295.

van Teijlingen, E., & Hundley, V. (2002). The importance of pilot studies. *Nursing Standard (Royal College of Nursing (Great Britain): 1987), 16*(40), 33–36. https://doi.org/10.7748/ns2002.06.16.40.33.c3214.

Vega, S., Marciscano, I., Holcomb, M., et al. (2013). Testing a top-down strategy for establishing a sustainable telemedicine program in a developing country: The Arizona telemedicine program–US Army–Republic of Panama initiative. *Telemedicine Journal and e-Health, 19*(10), 746–753. https://doi.org/10.1089/tmj.2013.0025.

Vilendrer, S., Patel, B., Chadwick, W., et al. (2020). Rapid deployment of inpatient telemedicine in response to COVID-19 across three health systems. *Journal of the American Medical Informatics Association: JAMIA, 27*(7), 1102–1109. https://doi.org/10.1093/jamia/ocaa077.

Warshaw, E. M., Hillman, Y. J., Greer, N. L., et al. (2011). Teledermatology for diagnosis and management of skin conditions: A systematic review. *Journal of the American Academy of Dermatology, 64*(4), 759–772. https://doi.org/10.1016/j.jaad.2010.08.026

Wootton, R. (2012). Twenty years of telemedicine in chronic disease management—an evidence synthesis. *Journal of Telemedicine and Telecare, 18*(4), 211–220. https://doi.org/10.1258/jtt.2012.120219

Yellowlees, P. M. (2005). Successfully developing a telemedicine system. *Journal of Telemedicine and Telecare, 11*(7), 331–335. https://doi.org/10.1258/135763305774472024

9

Social Determinants of Telehealth

Suzanne Goldenkranz, BA and Gil Addo, MBA

OBJECTIVES

1. Define the social determinants of telehealth.
2. Understand the implicit and explicit biases of providers when providing care via electronic modalities, and how those biases can affect healthcare outcomes.
3. Create awareness of health equity considerations in telehealth.

4. Explore considerations of patient needs when providing care virtually, including modalities of care, and broader patient needs.

CHAPTER OUTLINE

KEY TERMS

Social determinants of telehealth factors and conditions that contribute to a patient's success with telehealth. These include but are not limited to.

Infrastructure patients' access to the internet whether via broadband or other internet-enabled device

Housing patients must have a private and secure area to discuss confidential medical information

Devices patients must have the necessary devices, be educated in the use of technology, and understand the different forms of telehealth available to them

Cost consideration must be given to whether a patient has the resources to pay for telehealth visits (especially if outside of their current medical system), data limits on smartphones or other devices, or other constraints like the cost of high-speed internet in the home

Health literacy and education what can be done to make sure patients have the skills and understanding of their own health in order to make the most of their visits with providers?

Telehealth modalities different forms of telehealth used to best serve patients, including text communication, video visits, phone visits, and:

Chat bots AI-powered triage systems meant to assist in patient symptom checks, or provider understanding of patient needs

Remote patient monitoring technology used to transmit health information and biometrics from a patient in another setting (often home) to their provider (e.g., blood pressure cuffs, pulse oximeters, and blood glucose, weight, or temperature monitors)

eConsult asynchronous communication between providers regarding specific patient needs, looking for input or suggestions on how to better care for patients. Often primary care provider to specialty care provider, but can also be specialty care provider to other specialty care providers.

CASE STUDY: OHIO STATE UNIVERSITY

The Ohio State University (OSU), a large, urban, academic medical center and affiliated health system in the United States, provides over 1.8 million visits on an annual basis. A disproportionate amount of its patients (25%) are African American, and there are large numbers of other minority, poor, and homeless patients. Dr. Nwando Olayiwola serves as the Chair and Professor in the Department of Family and Community Medicine and has led its primary care use of telehealth, including expanding into additional areas of support for patients.

Telehealth began at OSU as a resource for underserved communities in the state of Ohio, starting with a large eConsult program for primary care providers to get specialty insights for individuals in carceral settings, who by nature of their incarceration have a hard time accessing care. The OSU program had grown over 10+ years to include virtual primary care and physician training to best serve the clinicians and help them understand how to use virtual care modalities in their practice even before the COVID-19 pandemic, which drove mass adoption of telehealth across other service lines and practice areas throughout the health system.

Building resources to address social determinants of health within telehealth practice has been a key learning and consideration for other providers as the center built a strong telehealth program. For example, understanding the challenges a particular patient may face in health or technology literacy, fear relating to their immigration status, housing, hearing or visual limitations, or preferred language can all inhibit the ability to serve a patient via telehealth and must be taken into consideration by providers. Additionally, OSU was able to use its local community partners to help ameliorate some of these social determinants of telehealth by providing trainings via local libraries for patients on how to do an eVisit, as well as having door-to-door trainers bring devices and set up internet in the homes of those without access, helping to bridge the digital divide for underserved populations in their backyard. This, coupled with additional provider training and resources, meant that patients were able to gain access to their local providers quickly and efficiently and build upon previous success of their telehealth work and keep patients engaged.

INTRODUCTION

The social determinants of health shown in Fig. 9.1 are conditions in the environments in which people are born, live, learn, work, play, worship, and age that affect a wide range of health, functioning, and quality-of-life outcomes and risks (US Office of Disease Prevention and Health Promotion, 2020; WHO, n.d.). These determinants create lasting inequality in healthcare access and can drive up to 80% of an individual's health outcomes (Manatt, 2019).

In the move to telehealth, there are additional factors and determinants that must be considered when working with patients from historically underserved communities. These social determinants of telehealth, and best practices for patients and providers to close gaps in healthcare, will be outlined in this chapter.

BACKGROUND

The impact of social determinants of health is well known in healthcare. There is a 48-year life expectancy spread across countries, attributed to factors outside of the individual (Marmot, 2005) but due to external conditions, and these factors have been linked with 80% of health outcomes (Manatt, 2019). These social determinants are defined as

external factors that lead to adverse health outcomes in defined populations. It is also well understood that these determinants can be impacted by targeting approaches to specific populations and groups, and by applying interventions and resources to these underserved populations (Solar & Irwin, 2010).

Telehealth took a meteoric growth path in 2020 as a result of the global COVID-19 pandemic. Around the world, telehealth limitations were quickly relaxed by governmental agencies as it became evident that this would be a way to reach patients quickly and easily, and resources were applied to encourage an expeditious switch to telehealth by providers (Fisk et al., 2020). Unfortunately, the use of telehealth was not evenly distributed across populations, and historically underserved communities were less likely to take advantage of these new resources (Weber et al., 2020).

By applying similar clinical understanding of how health outcomes and access are affected by external pressures, telehealth can be made to better fit those populations and individuals who need resources the most (Nouri et al., 2020). In order to create a more equitable telehealth practice, considerations must be made at both the provider and patient level for direct care, and at the policy level to best level the playing field for these types of services.

CASE STUDY: PETALUMA HEALTH CENTERS

Petaluma Health Centers (PHC), located in Northern California in ex-urban, suburban, and rural communities, serves 35,000–40,000 patients a year across a largely ethnic and racial minority population; about 50% of its patients are dual language speakers, and 31% are non–English-preferred patients. PHC, led by Dr. Danielle Oryn as CMO, has used telehealth in various modalities for many years to best provide resources, including specialty care, for its patients.

PHC has long used video visits within its clinics to connect patients to specialists who may not be accessible either in the community or without hardship to the patient (e.g., because of long travel times or lost work to get to an appointment); it also uses store-and-forward technology, especially for hard to come by visits like dermatology or ophthalmology. These specialist video visits with patients were also staffed by dual-cultural and dual-language Nurse Practitioners, Physician Assistants, or other care providers who would serve as translators and care navigators for patients, ensuring follow-up medications, appointments, labs, and so on would be ordered for the patient and that the patient understood all the health details being provided. This achieved a dual goal of ensuring both patient health literacy and strong patient care. Additional telehealth resources have also been utilized: a clinic for homeless patients, connecting providers with a patient and social worker on site to provide holistic patient care; a school site, where nurses or students could access primary care providers as needed; and even providing devices to patients released from inpatient stays to ensure easy access to primary care and their care team while recovering at home.

When the COVID-19 pandemic hit, PHC expanded its telehealth resources by adding specialist eConsults for primary care; this helped to keep its vulnerable patients out of clinical settings where they could be put more at risk of COVID-19 infection, but also ensured that patient care for chronic conditions was being continued.

During the COVID-19 pandemic, bilingual and bicultural front-end staff members were also redeployed to train patients on how to do a telehealth visit, as many patients who previously had been without a home internet-enabled device now had devices in their homes from schools because education had also gone virtual. Patients also were trained and assisted in the use of an online portal for form-filling and other administrative components of care. This training proved to be extremely effective, and telehealth training will continue to be part of the services PHC provides to its patients. Virtual translation services have also been rolled out for patients who need language support for a visit, either through a virtual AI device or through a third-party translator joining a visit to ensure that patients are able to receive care in their preferred language.

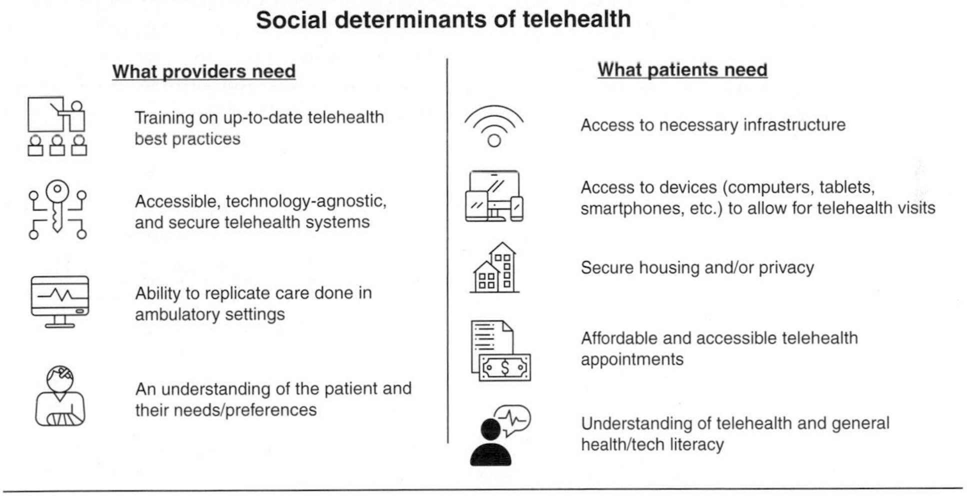

Social determinants of telehealth

What providers need

- Training on up-to-date telehealth best practices
- Accessible, technology-agnostic, and secure telehealth systems
- Ability to replicate care done in ambulatory settings
- An understanding of the patient and their needs/preferences

What patients need

- Access to necessary infrastructure
- Access to devices (computers, tablets, smartphones, etc.) to allow for telehealth visits
- Secure housing and/or privacy
- Affordable and accessible telehealth appointments
- Understanding of telehealth and general health/tech literacy

Fig. 9.1 Schema for social determinants of telehealth.

PROVIDERS

Considerations must start at the provider level before assuming that all patients in a panel are ready for best-practice telehealth; these considerations include both understanding the technological limitations and ensuring culturally competent care is provided for patients.

Marginalized communities such as African Americans in the United States (Kennedy et al., 2007) or Black, Asian, or Minority Ethnic communities in the United Kingdom (Burns, 2019) have had a long history of distrust of established medical systems, and these communities have had a similar historic distrust of or concerns with telehealth (George et al., 2012). Many of the same patient concerns can be found when they are asked about telehealth, including institutional racism, lack of culturally competent care, or access to services (George et al., 2012). However, when provided with telehealth options, 72% of Black, 69% of Asian, and 67% of Latinx survey respondents preferred telehealth to in-person visits with a provider, and 70% of Black and Asian respondents said these visits were easier to keep (California Pan-Ethnic Health Network, 2020). Culturally competent and accessible care must be provided in order to encourage these communities to access telehealth and make it available to all patients.

Culturally competent care can be defined as the "ability of systems to provide care to patients with diverse values, beliefs and behaviors, including tailoring delivery to meet patients' social, cultural, and linguistic needs" (Betancourt et al., 2002). This type of care should be foundational to medical practice, and multiple frameworks have been developed to build understanding and this competency for providers and for patients (Butler et al., 2016) in order to best serve diverse populations, including incorporating social determinants of health in patient care. This type of care and understanding must also be extended by providers into the telehealth ecosystem for the best patient outcomes and experiences.

Telehealth platforms should be easy for providers to access and bring into clinical practice, and considerations must be made of the ability to access the platform from any web-enabled **device** (computer, tablet, phone, etc.), rather than the platform being tied to a specific system or device (e.g., a computer in a clinic), in order to encourage adoption and ease of use. **Telehealth modalities** should also encourage easy communication with patients who may not be able to access specific types of applications due to service limitations or the level of technology available to them. Similarly, patient records and medical history, medications, and clinical notes must be available to providers regardless of location, and information must be shareable across disparate systems electronically and instantly through interoperability standards for providers working from different locations. This type of seamless communication can enable a provider to communicate and provide better care for a patient by reducing patient burden for their own health literacy and understanding, while giving the provider the resources to provide the best care for patients.

Providers must have access to telehealth platforms that are secure for both patients and providers and cannot be hacked or expose personal health information to other websites or individuals (Hofmann, 2020). This was an unfortunate issue in 2020's abrupt move to telehealth, as many safeguards and legal restrictions were relaxed to increase speedy adoptions, leading to exposed information, "Zoom bombings" (unwanted, generally malicious individuals showing up uninvited to video calls), and hacks of personal information, leading to lawsuits (Vielmetti, 2020). These types of interruptions can alter a patient's trust of telehealth and willingness to use these modalities for their healthcare.

Providers must also have ways to replicate care done in an ambulatory setting over telehealth, including reading patient vitals (temperature, blood pressure, etc.), and additional diagnostics that may take place in their care, such as blood work or other lab samples. These patient vitals are still important for care in the virtual setting, and thus there must be a way to get access to this kind of information. Private consumers in higher income brackets are more likely to purchase or utilize fitness trackers or smart wearable devices, and the digital divide across urban/suburban and rural areas also shows that adoption varies depending on the location of the user (Vogels, 2020), exacerbating the differences between communities. Next-generation tools and diagnostics such as **remote patient monitoring** devices (including wearables and fitness trackers), or even basic thermometers, should be made available to patients across all backgrounds in order to replicate these in-office tests, and patients need to be educated in how to take their own readings in conjunction with a provider or through asynchronous communication.

Providers must also be given access to additional resources for their own delivery of telehealth; for example, access to **eConsults** to streamline provider-to-provider communication and close access and education gaps in complex cases, and reduce the need for face-to-face patient care follow-up. eConsults specifically can reduce the need for in-person procedures, diagnostics, and testing by 45% (Reines et al., 2018); it follows that providing these resources to clinicians can drastically reduce patient face-to-face interactions. Patients also benefit from eConsults because the latter reduce the time and money that are associated with long wait times for specialty care, and avoid patients losing wages from missing work for an in-person visit. They are also used as a resource to bring specialty care into populations that have lower access to care, including undocumented patients who may be fearful of entering physical spaces due to their documentation status, rural patients or communities that may have to travel long distances to find high-quality specialists, or low-income patients without resources to visit specialty providers. These types of insights can also triage patients who do need care and teach providers how to best manage certain types of conditions through a virtual setting.

Providers must also take careful consideration of the patients they are encountering and provide culturally competent, patient-centered care. Patients come from a wide variety of racial and ethnic backgrounds and have diverse education and health literacy levels, with varying access to technology and infrastructure. Assessments for adequate virtual care require the comprehensive evaluation of patient-centered factors such as social support and community involvement, educational attainment, perceived challenges, health and digital literacy, and an analysis of what resources or understanding gaps there may be is vital to make sure a patient is receiving adequate care in a virtual setting. For example, an elderly patient coming from an underserved community or with a lack of formal health education may not have the health literacy to understand how to take their own pulse and will need to be taught these skills by community health workers or nurse advocates. Patient-centered care is not yet completely adapted in medical practice, and there is an opportunity to grow this model in general practice through telehealth.

Another factor to consider would be the patient's preferred language, and whether there is a need for translators as part of a video or telephone visit. Patients in any given setting, even in English-speaking countries, do not always come from households where English is the first language, and many inpatient visits and facilities include live translation services, printouts or materials in multiple languages, and even native language–speaking providers to assist in culturally competent care. In the United States, approximately two-thirds of hospitals provide some sort of translation services (Schiaffino et al., 2016), but those services may be limited to one or two languages, not covering the needs of all patients. Platforms and portals built in English without translations or resources for non-English-speaking patients have already been proven to be a resource inhibitor to access and can compound health hurdles for patients (Casillas et al., 2018) and create lack of utilization within English-limited communities. Many of the mass-adopted video visit systems in the United States were built with English as the primary language, without options for other languages in the portal, and with care being provided in English as the default, compounding the access challenges already felt in healthcare (Wetsman, 2020); 60% of patients with limited English proficiency reported that the telehealth they received was not in their preferred language (California Pan-Ethnic Health Network, 2020). Technology has evolved to allow for translators (often third parties) to join video or phone conversations and ensure that this barrier is lowered, but resources must be made available in advance of a visit with considerations for these patients; alternatively, AI systems like Google Translate can be brought into patient visits to assist in real time. Portals, monitoring devices, and other non-real systems must also come with instructions or resources in a patient's preferred language to ensure adoption and adherence.

PATIENTS

Patients will have a wide variety of external factors that will impact on whether or how telehealth can be delivered. These social determinants of telehealth will be laid out as factors to consider for patient care when deciding how best to serve patients from vulnerable and historically underserved communities where health outcomes are often the lowest. The social determinants of telehealth are:

1. infrastructure
2. housing
3. devices
4. cost
5. health literacy and education

This section will expand upon these social determinants of telehealth and provide clinical guidance on how to think about these areas when providing healthcare in a digital format to patients.

In order for a patient to access telehealth, they must actually have access to a device that can enable care delivery, as well as reliable or broadband internet access. Patients coming from different racial or ethnic backgrounds or economic strata, or those living with disabilities, will have varying access to these critical infrastructure needs for accessing telehealth. In the United States, the disparities in device and broadband internet access are quite stark when compared across different populations. Over 40% of respondents in the lowest income brackets (<$30,000 per year) reported they did not own a computer or have access to the internet, compared with nearly 100% of respondents with annual incomes of over $100,000 reporting that they had access to this technology (Anderson & Kumar, 2019). Individuals living with disabilities of any kind in the United States were nearly 20% less likely than individuals living without disabilities to have access to devices or internet (Perrin & Atske, 2021). Black or Latinx individuals were also significantly less likely to own a computer or have access to broadband than their white counterparts (Atske & Perrin, 2021). Without the fundamental infrastructure, video visits and app-based systems will not be able to reach the patients.

Cost for telehealth is another factor that will affect a patient's ability to access care, both in building programs and in the patient's ability to pay. Cost has been listed as the top barrier for healthcare systems to implement telehealth (Scott Kruse et al., 2018). Telehealth must be included in broadly accepted medical practice, and paid for at the same rates as traditional face-to-face visits. In the United States, the federally declared public health emergency during the 2020 COVID-19 pandemic established parity in telehealth payment and enabled telehealth to take off in practice by paying clinicians the same rate (Shachar et al., 2020) and reducing patient out-of-pocket expenses for care. Fee-for-service medicine, as is common in the

United States, serves as an additional barrier to telehealth adoption. Value-based care models have proved more effective in encouraging positive patient health outcomes, and telehealth is a way to ensure care for patients without having the additional burdens of transportation, wait times, or missed income, while still controlling chronic conditions and disease burdens (Cutter et al., 2020). Cost barriers must be reduced to encourage underserved populations to adopt telehealth.

Physical location is another factor that can contribute to a patient's ability to best use the telehealth available to them; this factor includes housing security and having established relationships with a local healthcare provider. In order to access telehealth visits, a patient must have a place that is private and quiet from which to access a video or telephone visit with a healthcare provider. Patients who live below the poverty line will have barriers to this type of location, and patients who are housing insecure or living with homelessness are less likely to have the ability to access providers electronically or take part in remote patient monitoring. Black, Asian, and Latinx individuals are also more likely to live in multigenerational or crowded households (Tareen, 2020), making private discussions and appointments much more difficult. If patients cannot access secure and private discussions with their healthcare provider, accommodations must be made such as encouraging a patient to find a quiet private location, or following up on sensitive information at a later time when they can be alone (e.g., sitting in their car during a lunch break, if they work in a crowded location). Patients who have a preferred healthcare provider must be able to continue those relationships through forms of telehealth, as patient-provider continuity has been attributed to lower mortality and higher patient satisfaction (Pereira Gray et al., 2018).

A patient's ability to use telehealth will also be limited by their understanding of telehealth itself as a field, the modalities, and what technologies are available to them. Care teams must give extra education to patients without understanding of how to use telehealth. Time must be allotted to ensure that patients are comfortable with these new forms of healthcare delivery, as was seen in 2020 by healthcare providers in the United States working with elderly patients (Ikram et al., 2020). These types of strategies include bringing patients' families into the care delivery process to help with the visits, providing practice visits for patients who are unfamiliar with new technology, and even providing one-click tablets for patients to streamline this process (Ikram et al., 2020).

Providers must also be willing to work with their patients to identify what the needs and limiting factors may be that are inhibiting telehealth adoption, and roll out solutions on a case-by-case basis. For example, dual-culture and -language nursing teams, or translators, can be brought in to help patients understand the goals of a telehealth visit or the process of remote patient monitoring, including teaching them how to use devices. Home care givers or family members can also be empowered, with patient consent, to assist in visits or with follow-up materials. Clinical social workers can also help to connect patients to resources like educational services, food delivery, or other resources that a visit reveals the patient may need, and can even help patients navigate difficulties with accessing and understanding care. Care teams have the unique ability to make sure patients are being supported throughout the virtual health delivery system as well as the in-person health delivery system.

The American Academy of Medical Colleges (AAMC) recently created a list of competencies for telehealth education to alleviate some of the lack of standardization. The guidelines are in six domains and include competencies for various levels of training, including physicians entering residency, recent graduates entering practice, and experienced faculty physicians (AAMC, 2021). Domain 2, Access and Equity in Telehealth, is relevant to addressing the social determinants of telehealth and is represented in the box below. The domain regarding access and equity in telehealth is to guide physician trainees to promote equitable access to care, by understanding telehealth delivery that addresses and mitigates cultural biases as well as physician bias for or against telehealth and that accounts for physical and mental disabilities and non-health-related individual and community needs and limitations (AAMC, 2021).

AAMC Telehealth Competencies Domain 2: Access and Equity in Telehealth

Entering residency	Entering practice (recent residency graduate)	Experienced faculty physician (3–5 years post-residency)
1a. Describes one's own implicit and explicit biases and their implications when considering telehealth	1b. Describes and mitigates one's own implicit and explicit biases during telehealth encounters	1c. Role models and teaches how to recognize and mitigate biases during telehealth encounters

AAMC Telehealth Competencies Domain 2: Access and Equity in Telehealth—cont'd

Entering residency	Entering practice (recent residency graduate)	Experienced faculty physician (3–5 years post-residency)
2a. Defines how telehealth can affect health equity and mitigate or amplify gaps in access to care	2b. Leverages technology to promote health equity and mitigate gaps in access to care	2c. Promotes and advocates the use of telehealth to promote health equity and access to care and to advocate for policy change in telehealth to reduce inequities
3a. When considering telehealth, assesses the patient's needs, preferences, access to, and potential cultural, social, physical, cognitive, and linguistic and other communication barriers to technology use	3b. When considering telehealth, accommodates the patient's needs, preferences, and potential cultural, social, physical, cognitive, and linguistic and communication barriers to technology use	3c. When considering telehealth, role models how to advocate for improved access to it and accommodates the patient's needs, preferences, and potential cultural, social, physical, cognitive, and linguistic and communication barriers to technology use

AAMC. (2021). *Telehealth competencies across the learning continuum.* AAMC New and Emerging Areas in Medicine Series. Washington, DC: AAMC.

KEY POINTS

- Providers must take considerations of telehealth modality and individual patient circumstances into account when operating in a digital environment.
- Social determinants of telehealth can affect how and where telehealth can be used with patients, as well as outcomes from these types of care.

- Telehealth can either bridge health equity gaps or exacerbate existing issues based on how it is applied or utilized.

ACKNOWLEDGMENT

Additional thank you to Dr. Danielle Oryn and Dr. Nwando Olayiwola for their interviews and sharing their expertise in clinical rollouts of telehealth.

？ CRITICAL THINKING QUESTIONS

1. What are the Social Determinants of Telehealth?
2. How does a patient's social determinants affect their access to telehealth?
3. What are 3 ways you can ensure your telehealth practice incorporates access for all patients?

REFERENCES

AAMC. (2021). *Telehealth competencies across the learning Continuum. AAMC New and Emerging Areas in Medicine Series.* Washington, DC: AAMC.

Anderson, M., & Kumar, M. (2019). *Digital divide persists even as lower-income Americans make gains in tech adoption.* Pew Research Center. https://www.pewresearch.org/fact-tank/2019/05/07/digital-divide-persists-even-as-lower-income-americans-make-gains-in-tech-adoption/. [Accessed 1 November 2021].

Atske, S., & Perrin, A. (2021). *Home Broadband Adoption, computer ownership vary by race, ethnicity in the U.S.* Pew Research Center. https://www.pewresearch.org/fact-tank/2021/07/16/home-broadband-adoption-computer-ownership-vary-by-race-ethnicity-in-the-u-s/. [Accessed 30 January, 2022].

Betancourt, J. R., Green, A. R., & Carrillo, J. E. (2002). *Cultural competence in health care: Emerging frameworks and practical approaches.* New York: The Commonwealth Fund.

Burns, R. (2019). *Medecins du Monde's (MdM) 2019 Observatory Report Left Behind: The state of Universal healthcare coverage.* MHADRI. https://mhadri.org/2019/12/17/medecins-du-mondes-mdm-2019-observatory-report-left-behind-the-state-of-universal-healthcare-coverage/. [Accessed 17 December 2020].

Butler, M., McCreedy, E., Schwer, N., et al. (2016). *Improving cultural competence to reduce health disparities.* (Comparative Effectiveness reviews, No. 170.) table 21, cultural competence models. Rockville (MD): Agency for Healthcare Research and Quality (US). https://www.ncbi.nlm.nih.gov/books/NBK361115/table/ch5.t1/. [Accessed 1 November 2021].

California Pan-Ethnic Health Network. (2020). Equity in the age of telehealth: Considerations for California policymakers. https://cpehn.org/updates/2020/12/equity-age-telehealth-considerations-california-policymakers.

Casillas, A., Moreno, G., Grotts, J., et al. (2018). A digital language divide? The relationship between internet medication refills and medication adherence among limited English proficient (LEP) patients. *Journal of Racial and Ethnic Health Disparities, 5*(6), 1373–1380. https://doi.org/10.1007/s40615-018-0487-9.

Cutter, C., Berlin, N., & Fendrick, A. M. (2020). *Establishing a value-based 'new normal' for telehealth: Health Affairs Blog.* Health Affairs. https://www.healthaffairs.org/do/10.1377/hblog20201006.638022/full/. [Accessed 1 November 2021].

Fisk, M., Livingstone, A., & Pit, S. W. (2020). Telehealth in the context of COVID-19: Changing perspectives in Australia, the United Kingdom, and the United States. *Journal of Medical Internet Research, 22*(6), e19264. https://doi.org/10.2196/19264.

George, S., Hamilton, A., & Baker, R. S. (2012). How do low-income urban African Americans and Latinos feel about telemedicine? A diffusion of innovation analysis. *International Journal of Telemedicine and Applications 2012*, 715194. https://doi.org/10.1155/2012/715194.

Hofmann, L. (2020). *Is Zoom GDPR Compliant? (Video Conferencing tools & data Protection risks).* Pridatect. https://www.pridatect.co.uk/zoom-gdpr-compliant/. [Accessed 1 November 2021].

Ikram, U., Gallani, S., Figueroa, J. F., et al. (2020). *4 Strategies to make telehealth work for elderly patients.* Harvard Business Review. https://hbr-org.cdn.ampproject.org/c/s/hbr.org/amp/2020/11/4-strategies-to-make-telehealth-work-for-elderly-patients. [Accessed 1 November 2021].

Kennedy, B. R., Mathis, C. C., & Woods, A. K. (2007). African Americans and their distrust of the health care system: Healthcare for diverse populations. *Journal of Cultural Diversity, 14*(2), 56–60.

Koonin, L. M., Hoots, B., Tsang, C. A., et al. (2020). Trends in the use of telehealth during the emergence of the COVID-19 pandemic — United States, January–March 2020. *MMWR Morbidity and Mortality Weekly Report, 69*, 1595–1599. https://doi.org/10.15585/mmwr.mm6943a3.

Manatt, P., & Phillips, L. L. P. (2019). *Medicaid's role in addressing social determinants of health.* RWJF. https://www.rwjf.org/en/library/research/2019/02/medicaid-s-role-in-addressing-social-determinants-of-health.html.

Nouri, S., Khoong, E. C., Lyles, C. R., et al. (2020). Addressing equity in telemedicine for chronic disease management during the COVID-19 pandemic. *NEJM Catalyst Innovations in Care Delivery, 1*(3). https://catalyst.nejm.org/doi/full/10.1056/CAT.20.0123.

Pereira Gray, D. J., Sidaway-Lee, K., White, E., et al. (2018). Continuity of care with doctors-a matter of life and death? A systematic review of continuity of care and mortality. *BMJ Open, 8*(6), e021161. https://doi.org/10.1136/bmjopen-2017-021161.

Perrin, A., & Atske, S. (2021). *Americans with disabilities less likely than those without to own some digital devices.* Pew Research Center. https://www.pewresearch.org/fact-tank/2021/09/10/americans-with-disabilities-less-likely-than-those-without-to-own-some-digital-devices/. [Accessed 30 January 30, 2022].

Reines, C., Miller, L., Olayiwola, J. N., et al. (2018). Can eConsults save Medicaid? *NEJM Catalyst, 4*(4).

Schiaffino, M. K., Nara, A., & Mao, L. (2016). Language services in hospitals vary by ownership and location. *Health Affairs (Project Hope), 35*(8), 1399–1403. https://doi.org/10.1377/hlthaff.2015.0955.

Scott Kruse, C., Karem, P., Shifflett, K., et al. (2018). Evaluating barriers to adopting telemedicine worldwide: A systematic review. *Journal of Telemedicine and Telecare, 24*(1), 4–12. https://doi.org/10.1177/1357633X16674087.

Shachar, C., Engel, J., & Elwyn, G. (2020). Implications for telehealth in a postpandemic future: Regulatory and privacy issues. *Journal of the American Medical Association, 323*(23), 2375–2376. https://doi.org/10.1001/jama.2020.7943.

Solar, O., & Irwin, A. (2010). A conceptual framework for action on the social determinants of health. *Social Determinants of Health Discussion Paper 2 (Policy and Practice).* Geneva, Switzerland: World Health Organization.

Tareen, S. (2020). *Coronavirus complicates safety for families living together.* ABC News. https://abcnews.go.com/US/wireStory/correction-virus-outbreak-multigenerational-families-story-70648439. [Accessed 1 November 2021].

US Office of Disease Prevention and Health Promotion. (2020). *Social determinants of health.* https://www.healthypeople.gov/2020/topics-objectives/topic/social-determinants-of-health. [Accessed 1 November 2021].

Vielmetti, B. (2020). *Lawsuit: Zoom security failings exposed confidential medical information.* Milwaukee Journal Sentinel. https://www.jsonline.com/story/news/local/milwaukee/2020/04/17/lawsuit-zoom-security-failings-exposed-confidential-medical-information/2982350001/. [Accessed 1 November 2021].

Vogels, E. A. (2020). *About one-in-five Americans use a smart watch or fitness tracker.* Pew Research Center. https://www.pewresearch.org/fact-tank/2020/01/09/about-one-in-five-americans-use-a-smart-watch-or-fitness-tracker/. [Accessed 1 November 2021].

Weber, E., Miller, S. J., Astha, V., et al. (2020). Characteristics of telehealth users in NYC for COVID-related care during the coronavirus pandemic. *Journal of the American Medical Informatics Association: JAMIA, 27*(12), 1949–1954. https://doi.org/10.1093/jamia/ocaa216.

Wetsman, N. (2020). *Telehealth wasn't designed for non-English speakers.* https://www.theverge.com/21277936/telehealth-english-systems-disparities-interpreters-online-doctor-appointments. [Accessed 1 November 2021].

World Health Organization. (n.d.). *Social determinants of health.* https://www.who.int/health-topics/social-determinants-of-health. [Accessed 1 November 2021].

10

Inclusive Innovation

Brooke Ellison, PhD, MPP

> *"We have the Internet of Everything but not the inclusion of everyone."*
>
> **Ajaypal Singh Banga**

OBJECTIVES

1. Describe how technology affects the lives of people with disabilities.
2. Perceive how people with disabilities experience health challenges and health disparities.
3. Articulate the ways through which telehealth might help to address disability-related health challenges.
4. Define the term "inclusive innovation" and what it means for telehealth.
5. Determine the need for inclusion of people with disabilities in technology and telehealth.

CHAPTER OUTLINE

KEY TERMS

Activities of daily living a term used to collectively describe fundamental skills required to independently care for oneself, such as eating, bathing, and mobility

Assistive technology products, equipment, and systems that enhance learning working and daily living for persons with disabilities

Disability a physical or mental condition that limits a person's movements, senses, or activities

Disability associated health expenditures additional health-care costs related to injury, diseases, and chronic conditions associated with disability

Health disparity Health disparities are preventable differences in the burden of disease, injury, violence, or opportunities to achieve optimal health that are experienced by socially disadvantaged populations

Inclusion the practice or policy of providing equal access to opportunities and resources for people who might otherwise be excluded or marginalized, such as those who have physical or mental disabilities and members of other minority groups

Inclusive innovation technological development in telehealth, where those with disabilities and caregivers are seen as strategic partners

Secondary health conditions "any additional physical or mental health condition that occurs as a result of having a primary disabling condition

Universal design the design and composition of an environment so that it can be accessed, understood and used to the greatest extent possible by all

INTRODUCTION

Telehealth is a promising modality for providing healthcare and healthcare access to communities historically underserved by the medical apparatus. Telehealth is thought to be a mechanism by which to bridge barriers that often impede access to care. One population that systematically and repeatedly encounters barriers to care but whose healthcare needs are among the most involved are people with disabilities. For many reasons, people with disabilities have largely been underexplored as a public health group experiencing health disparities, but there is a specific definition of "health disparity" in the public health literature which refers to "differences in health outcomes at the population level, that these differences are linked to a history of social, economic, or environmental disadvantages, and that these differences are regarded as avoidable" (Krahn et al., 2015). Individuals from racial and ethnic minorities have long been the subjects of health disparities research, and deservedly so. Because of work done in this field, strategic and policy-driven efforts have been made to begin to reduce the impact of these disparities. However, as people with disabilities have not regularly been thought of as a minority group experiencing significant health inequities resulting from a history of injustice, ameliorative efforts largely have not been taken to address these social inequities for the disabled population. The health disparities experienced by people with disabilities are vast and vary considerably in type. People with disabilities experience health disparities as they relate to healthcare access, manifestations and health behaviors, prevalence of disease, and social determinants of health (see Chapter 9). These present a multifaceted and extraordinarily complex image of health disparity that complicates the lives of people with disabilities.

People with disabilities often have difficulty gaining access to facility-based healthcare appointments, despite the fact that they can require ongoing healthcare. The reasons are multifaceted and manifold, depending on circumstances and individual need. Accessibility is a challenge for people with disabilities in any aspect of social life, and this is no less (and sometimes even more) the case in a healthcare setting. The establishment of telehealth videoconferences and remote patient monitoring systems can potentially alleviate the burden that access barriers create for people with disabilities. As Young and Edwards note, "this is especially true for people who live in remote and underserved areas, or have difficulty leaving their home or getting to the doctor's office." Young & Edwards (2020). The benefits of telehealth are also apparent when it comes to accessing care from medical specialists who can sometimes be at a distance, improved patient satisfaction, and an overall reduction in emergency department utilization. When telehealth applications are crafted correctly and planned comprehensively, the benefits of many of them can neatly meet the needs of people with disabilities.

DISABILITY AND HEALTH

As Chaet et al. (2017) state, the advances of telehealth technologies provide new channels through which to access care, as well as opportunities for truly patient-centered care. However, at the same time, the advancements of telehealth and telemedicine have not developed with inclusion in mind, and might also exacerbate familiar vulnerabilities and disparities seen in the healthcare system. People with disabilities, like other groups historically underrepresented in the healthcare apparatus, face particular healthcare challenges that can either be improved or exacerbated by advancements in telehealth. We begin this chapter by exploring some of the healthcare challenges particularly experienced by people with disabilities, and how these disparities might be addressed through telehealth innovation.

Health Access

Healthcare access, or healthcare accessibility, refers to an individual's ability to take part in the healthcare system without financial, geographic, or institutionalized barriers. "Disability" is a broad term with many manifestations. According to the WHO, it has three dimensions: (1) impairment in body function or structure, such as loss of a limb or loss of vision; (2) limitation in activity, such as difficulty seeing, hearing, walking, or problem-solving; and (3) restriction in ability and normal daily activities. This constellation of dimensions relates directly to an individual's ability to experience and access the environment when transportation or architectural accessibility is not established. Access to healthcare is one of the most significant—yet likely most avoidable—manifestations of disparity experienced by people with disabilities. Access to healthcare, or lack thereof, can take the form of physical barriers, such as stairs, communication barriers, illegible websites, and discriminatory policies (CDC, 2013). The functional effects of these physical barriers are significant. For instance, in the United States, an investigation of 2400 primary care facilities serving Medicaid patients in California highlighted that fewer than half of the facilities were fully accessible (i.e., equipped with ramps for entry, wide doorways, and accessible bathrooms). Far fewer of these treatment facilities had medical examination equipment that was usable or adequate for people with disabilities.

In many ways, advances in telehealth and telemedicine can democratize and broaden access to healthcare. Telehealth and telemedicine circumvent the need for transportation in the pursuit of needed healthcare services, as well as the need for an attendant or caregiver. What is more, the access to healthcare via telemedicine encounters also obviates the need, at least in many cases, for a patient to visit an inaccessible clinician's office, a barrier which would otherwise prevent the receipt of care. From this vantage point, telehealth and telemedicine could revolutionize the degree of access that many people with disabilities encounter when they attempt to access healthcare.

However, particularly when considering people with disabilities, telemedicine might not be the right healthcare delivery mechanism, unless it is crafted and implemented in a way that is complementary to the needs of this population. In the referral, implementation, and design of telemedicine strategies, it is incumbent upon clinicians and healthcare providers to determine the appropriate mechanism of care delivery for members of this population, through a process that takes into consideration resources, technological aptitude, differences in culture, and differences in ability. The challenges associated with healthcare access that are experienced by people with disabilities make this population particularly well-suited for reaping the benefits of telemedicine applications, but the realization of these benefits can only take place when this population is included in the technological design.

Health Outcomes

People with disabilities are at risk of experiencing secondary health conditions that occur following the onset of disability. According to the WHO's World Report on Disability (WIIO, 2011), people with disabilities are far more likely to experience depression, chronic pain, and osteoporosis. These secondary conditions are particular risks for people with conditions such as cerebral palsy, spina bifida, postpolio paralysis, and spinal cord injury. While people with disabilities develop the very same health challenges that affect those without disability, they are also more susceptible to developing chronic conditions as a result of behaviors and sequelae associated with their disability, such as limited physical activity, cardiovascular disease, and type 2 diabetes. For instance, as the WHO noted, people with disabilities have a greater susceptibility to age-related conditions at an earlier age, as many of them experience the aging process earlier or at a more accelerated pace than people without disabilities. For instance, some people with developmental disabilities demonstrate significant signs of aging in their 40s and 50s and, as a result, may experience a far earlier onset of such age-related conditions as Alzheimer disease, dementia, loss of strength and balance, and osteoporosis. In addition, the health-related behaviors practiced by people with disabilities—for reasons beyond their own

control—can be vastly different than those of people without disabilities. As an investigation in Australia indicated, people with disabilities aged 15–64 years were more likely to be overweight or obese than nondisabled people and were far more likely to be physically inactive due, in large part, to mobility limitations. (Keramat et al. 2021).

Other behavioral health risks demonstrated to affect people with disabilities disproportionately include smoking, alcohol consumption, drug use, and depression. There is also a more unexpected health disparity: exposure to violence and sexual abuse appears to disproportionately affect disabled individuals. Accompanying these risks of violence is a higher risk of unintentional injury by traffic accidents, burns, falls, and accidents related to assistive devices (WHO 2011). All of these generate significant disparities when it comes to health outcomes in healthcare access, and result in a higher risk of premature death among individuals with disabilities.

The steps taken to address the health disparities experienced by people with disabilities have been notably meager, with most attention being given to disability prevention rather than addressing existing health challenges that exist, such as barriers to access and maintenance of chronic conditions. In order for reform efforts to be comprehensive, they must address the three prongs of healthcare: access, affordability, and quality. For people with disabilities, obtaining each of these three prongs of healthcare can be difficult. Access can be a particular challenge, with disability affecting patients' ability to navigate transportation and architecture; disability is highly correlated with poverty, thereby reducing affordability; and disability sometimes creates secondary health conditions that disproportionately affect the quality of the healthcare patients receive.

The advancements of telehealth are particularly well suited for the management of chronic healthcare conditions. Many chronic healthcare conditions and sequelae associated with health behaviors can be managed quite easily via remote encounters. While disability and chronic conditions, as well as disability and behavioral health conditions, can often go hand in hand, the opportunity to fully address and alleviate the consequences of these relationships is wholly contingent on the ability of people with disabilities to access the technology that supports telehealth and telemedicine innovation.

DISABILITY AND TECHNOLOGY

The role that technology plays in the lives of people with disabilities cannot be overstated. In fact, one could argue that it is impossible to talk about disability without also talking about technology. In a new era of inclusion and innovation, the reverse should also be the case.

Technology and Independent Living

Many people with disabilities of all kinds live at home in their communities. For instance, according to data collected by SCI-Info, 87% of people with paralysis (either quadriplegia or paraplegia) are discharged from the hospital to their homes (SCI-Info, n.d.). In order for community-dwelling people with disability to live at home in a fully participatory way, technology must be developed that provides these citizens with modalities to interact with their environments. As Chen et al. (2007) noted, people who live with disabilities are increasingly reliant on electronic devices to improve their ability to interact with appliances and environmental controls.

Even for people with complex disabilities, there is an array of modalities by which to operate devices. However, as Folan et al. (2015) argue, we live in an age in which computers and interactive devices play an increasingly prominent role in our everyday lives, and technologies that were useful in the past have not kept pace with current technology demands, especially in telehealth and telemedicine. While meaningful quality of life improvements and a social participation can be established post-injury through adaptive and assistive technologies (Folan et al., 2015), all efforts must be made to explore additional, and even intersectional, strategies by which to maximize interactions between people with disabilities and technology.

Assistive Technologies and Quality of Life

It has been demonstrated in repeated studies that assistive technology, and specifically technology that can provide computer access, has a positive association with quality of life for people with disabilities. Baldassin et al. (2018) conducted a literature review to assess the relationship between assistive technology use and quality of life for people with spinal cord injury. As these researchers write, spinal cord injury compromises an individual's ability to perform activities of daily living (ADLs), which negatively affects their quality of life. As estimates of quality of life are associated with meeting personal needs, controlling one's environment, and having the autonomy to make personal decisions about one's life, assistive technology devices for technology, like the computer, can provide "one of the few possibilities for access to information, social networks, work, and leisure activities, thereby improving the perception of efficacy and greater autonomy" (Baldassin et al., 2018).

The World Health Organization has defined "quality of life" as personal perceptions of an individual's position in life in the context of the cultural and value systems in which they live and in relation to their goals, expectations, standards, and concerns (WHO, 1995). The need to maximize quality of life applies to all people with disabilities, and the maximization of quality of life is intricately tied to health and wellness, as well as to inclusion in technology that promotes health and wellness.

DISABILITY AND TELEHEALTH

Telehealth and telemedicine are well designed to address health disparities brought about by challenges in healthcare access, social determinants of health, and sociobehavioral health conditions. These are the types of healthcare challenges that people with disabilities often confront. For these reasons, the 15 million people with disabilities in the United States represent a critical population for whom to develop and implement telehealth solutions.

People with disabilities often have complex medical needs and healthcare access disparities for which telehealth and digital health are particularly well suited, and yet these very same people are among the least likely to have access to those technologies. Telehealth not only brings episodic connectivity between patients and their clinicians but may also prevent the burden of secondary conditions through chronic monitoring. According to the WHO, disability leads to greater susceptibility to developing chronic conditions as a result of behaviors and sequelae associated with disability (WHO, 2011). The utilization of telehealth applications for healthcare monitoring provides protection from iatrogenic exposure to infectious agents. Virtual healthcare can enhance access and improve quality of care, especially when optimized through remote patient monitoring and virtual video visits, which reduce the need for on-site visits that can be both physically and financially burdensome for members of this population.

For people with disabilities, technology has the potential to provide an existence with reduced adverse health outcomes, reduced care coordination needs, and a reduced risk of long-term hospitalization or institutionalization. But achieving these goals means changing the way medicine is practiced. The advancement of telehealth for everyone, but especially for people with disabilities, requires influencing evidence-based guidelines, facilitating large clinical trials, and providing health services without the health system as intermediary. In all circumstances, persons with disabilities should be engaged in technological development, innovation, clinical trial design and participation, and consumer experience reporting and testing. Powerful collaborations of patients, health centers, and industry will help create an equal partnership in technological innovation and adoption.

The health disparities that people with disabilities face are coupled with social disparities that make the treatment of these health disparities that much more difficult. Advances in telehealth and telemedicine will have to meet both of these needs. According to the Pew Research Center, Americans with disabilities are considerably less likely to ever go online. When the internet provides the most immediate medium to establish communication between physicians and patients, this technological disparity can be the basis of a concomitant health disparity. What is more, people with disabilities are 20% less likely than people without disabilities to own a computer, smartphone, or tablet—the mechanisms by which much telehealth innovation is delivered and telehealth information is recorded (Anderson & Perrin, 2021). Understanding the ways that people with disabilities do or do not have access to even the most basic technologies—hearing directly from them regarding the barriers they face and what is needed to overcome these barriers—is imperative.

INCLUSIVE INNOVATION

The growth of digital health and telehealth technologies lies at the forefront of medicine and the center of innovation,

---

CASE 1

THRIVE Services uses assistive technology in the care of its residents, most of whom have physical or developmental disabilities. THRIVE has invested in assistive technology devices and plans since it came into existence decades ago, and these initiatives started with simple, low-tech solutions that have grown in complexity over the years.

In its early stages, THRIVE used relatively simple yet novel technology, such as adapted switches, to help allow people with disabilities to live their lives more independently and to meet their needs and daily life goals. In the years since, THRIVE has continued to develop the technology it has utilized. Central to this development was gaining the insights of people with disabilities, in terms of what they need and how they would like to use technology.

THRIVE wanted to make its facility more "accessible" and, as a result, provide greater access to its residents. Accessibility meant more than just wide doorways and open spaces; THRIVE also wanted residents to be able to meaningfully engage with their environment. However, understanding where the limitations lay required deep, engaged conversations and observations of people with disabilities in their environments, and documenting of their experiences, so that the technology implemented was, indeed, technology that could be used meaningfully.

One of the residents at THRIVE whose experiences were particularly helpful was Evelyn, a 35-year-old woman with cerebral palsy. Evelyn is smart, talented, and a burgeoning author; however, her disability and lack of access to technology was making it difficult for her to utilize and build upon her talents. This level of inaccessibility was a good source of frustration. After speaking with administrators at THRIVE, the organization was able to apply for a grant to purchase computer access equipment for Evelyn to allow her to connect with her world more effectively.

---

and has, perhaps, the biggest potential marginal impact on the lives of people with disabilities. Yet participation from people with disabilities in this world of technological innovation remains woefully limited, despite the impact it can have on their quality of life, thereby leaving them behind in this medical and technological shift. The future of medicine and telehealth that emerges through the current technological revolution, together with societal advancement, should reflect a new era of accessibility and inclusion in which people with disabilities are seen as valuable and strategic partners who serve alongside the medical community and technology sector to develop innovation. This is truly inclusive for a population whose needs have often been overlooked but whose knowledge and experience might prove invaluable.

Despite the lack of access to technology that many people with disabilities face, there is a deep commitment among these individuals to be a part of the current healthcare technological revolution. For instance, as Noel and Ellison (2020) demonstrated, people with disabilities accounted for 65% (58,406) of beneficiaries using telehealth. People with disabilities used over 66% (182,858) of all telehealth services. Between 2014 and 2016, there was a 37.7% increase in the number of beneficiaries with disabilities using telehealth, and a 53.7% increase in the total services these beneficiaries used (Center for Medicare and Medicaid Services, 2018). In addition, in situations in which initiatives have been undertaken to increase technological inclusivity for people with disabilities, there has been a strong adoption of these innovations. To be sure, people with disabilities are ideal candidates both from whom to glean insights regarding their technology-based experiences and for whom the advances of telehealth might provide the biggest marginal benefit. However, people with disabilities are not only consumers of medicine and healthcare; they are consumers of technology to maximize their quality of life, like most others.

Telehealth and technology must have an ongoing strategy of inclusion of everyone. It is unsurprising that what is beneficial for people with disabilities also turns out to be beneficial for everyone. The concept of *universal design* is built off of this very idea. Universal design has been defined as "the design and composition of an environment so that it can be accessed, understood, and used: (1) to the greatest possible extent; (2) in the most independent and natural manner possible; (3) in the widest possible range of situations; and (4) without the need of adaptation, modification, assistive devices, or specialized solutions by any persons of any age or size or having any particular physical, sensory, mental health, or intellectual disability."[1] However, while universal design often typically applies to architecture and the built environment, it can also apply to technology. In fact, an additional definition offered for universal design

---

[1]This definition has been excerpted from the Irish Disability Act of 2005.

is, "in relation to electronic systems, any electronics-based process of creating products, services, or systems so that they may be used by any person" (Centre for Excellence in Universal Design, 2020). In other words, when it comes to the advancement of technological innovation, a design that is optimal is a design that accommodates the needs of many, but especially people who require alternative means of access. What is good for this population is often good for everyone.

Major stakeholders in the technology sector have only just begun to realize and learn from the experiences of people with disabilities, and their innovation has accelerated as a result. As the market of devices that utilize technology historically used by people with disabilities has grown and has included the general population, more capacity has been generated for enhanced, advanced innovation that benefits everyone. Table 10.1 discusses technologies that have involved the development of increased interfaces through which people with disabilities can engage with technology (Jones et al., 2008; Reimer-Reiss & Wacker, 2000; Rigby et al., 2011). Data and studies have indicated the overall

TABLE 10.1	Different Technologies
Technology	**Description**
Age-tech	Technology that is designed to meet the needs of an aging population (Woods, 2019)
Euphonia	Personalized speech recognition for nonstandard speech (Choney, 2019; Emanuel, 2020)
Project DIVA	Google Assistant accessibility (Caggioni, 2019)

benefit of implementing inclusion in the innovation process. However, it is now time to scale these innovations through greater involvement from the private sector.

The vision of inclusion makes sense from many vantage points. There is a strong moral imperative for "inclusive innovation": we, as a society, are better off when everyone can take part in it and our societal developments must take place in a way that reflects that belief. People with disabilities, in particular, have historically been removed from social conversations in general and from technology-related conversations specifically, and this has led to a technological frontier that has been largely absent of the voices, insights, and experiences of people with disabilities.

In addition to the humanitarian importance of inclusive innovation, designing technology to meet the needs of people with disabilities also makes sound financial sense. The global disability market is sizable, representing 1.3 billion people worldwide with a projected $1.2 trillion in annual disposable income (Brodey, 2019). Especially given our aging population who will experience disability at a greater prevalence, innovations for people with disabilities have a large economic and political potential that promises significant returns on investment (Donovan, 2016). Considering technologies like the Amazon Alexa and Google Home Assistant, in a framework that mirrors the societal benefits of universal design, what is useful for people with disabilities is also often useful for most others.

Now is the time for technology innovators of all kinds—telehealth, telemedicine, and more generalized technology, alike—to seize upon this intersection of need, demand, and opportunity. Given the divide between the state of technological innovation and how it is used by people with disabilities, there is tremendous potential for a mutually beneficial collaboration between people with disabilities, tech giants, and smaller technological innovators. The current climate is optimal for social entrepreneurship, in which industry and disability advocates unite to research and develop in a way that involves everyone: true inclusive innovation.

CASE 2

Noah is a seven-year-old boy who has cystic fibrosis. Noah is highly social, extremely active, loves his friends and family, but is at chronic risk of respiratory infection that could bring about significant complications for him. When Noah was preparing for second grade, it became clear to his parents that he needed to remain outside of a hospital setting as much as possible but that he needed ongoing care from his doctors in order to stay healthy.

When Noah contracted pneumonia and required IV antibiotics to treat it, his parents were concerned that he would have to be admitted to the hospital. Noah's pulmonologist, however, discussed with them the possibility of Noah remaining at home, under their care, but with close monitoring by his doctors through a remote patient monitoring system. Through a monitoring system implemented by the hospital's IT department, Noah could have his breathing monitored through a Bluetooth-enabled stethoscope, he could have his oxygen saturations under the oversight of his pulmonologist through a Bluetooth-enabled pulse oximeter, and he could have his temperature and pulse monitored using a pairing thermometer. What is more, through the portal that the remote patient monitoring included, Noah's parents could remain in regular contact with his physicians, uploading vital signs and data on a regular basis, sending portal messages as numbers changed in either a positive or negative direction. It was through this system that Noah could recover from pneumonia safely at home, under the care of his parents.

INCLUSION: HOW TO DO IT

While many technologies hold promise for independence and community-based living for people with severe disability, engineers designing these technologies must be aware of the contexts of individuals' experiences, challenges, perspectives, and beliefs within which the technologies will be used. Human factors researchers and practitioners have developed a well-established framework for including these factors in product and process design, known as the Systems Engineering Initiative for Patient Safety (SEIPS). SEIPS 2.0 is an extension of one of the most well-regarded human factors systems models used in healthcare, the SEIPS model (Carayon et al., 2006; Holden et al., 2013). The approach of these models captures the social influences, cognitive processes, perceived ease of use, usefulness and actual use of new technology (Davis et al., 1989; Venkatesh & Davis., 2000) that affect community engagement and functional independence.

Now is an unprecedented time in all aspects of life. The healthcare crisis precipitated by COVID-19 has changed the way people from all parts of the world live their lives. The practice of medicine is, perhaps, more significantly affected than any other facet of daily life, and the centrality of telehealth and telemedicine to the new landscape of medicine cannot be overstated. Telehealth and telemedicine must advance to meet the growing demand, but they must advance comprehensively. Realizing the future trajectory of medicine, tech giants like Google, Microsoft, and Amazon have entered the telehealth space, joining smaller technology innovators who have paved the path as this field has grown. Now, more than ever, there is immeasurable enthusiasm around and support for rapid innovation in telehealth and telemedicine to meet the demands of an aging, and therefore increasingly disabled, population requiring healthcare. Yet the advancement of these areas of innovation has largely been absent of the voices, insights, and needs of people with disabilities. The future of telemedicine and telehealth relies on innovation—not simply innovation, but inclusive innovation.

Inclusion in innovation must begin at the idea-generation phase. It is arguably less that the telehealth and telemedicine innovators are unaware of or unresponsive to the fact that people with disabilities have needs than that they are unclear about what these needs are and how they affect lives in practical ways. This divide between innovation and the lived experiences of people with disabilities is the fulcrum of this social disparity, and visionaries in healthcare and technology can bridge this divide as the field moves forward through inclusion of the disabled voice. Realizing the full promise of inclusive innovation is contingent on collaborations that put the user at the center: to learn from, to be guided by, and to test on behalf of.

Though the voices of people with disabilities have been removed from many technological advances, the promotion of deep and comprehensive engagement within the disability community can lead to diversity of experience in the idea-generation phase of innovation. In order to know what people with disabilities experience, and therefore what they need, all efforts must be made to incorporate their knowledge into conversations surrounding the planning and execution of research and development agendas in technology. It is important to isolate and identify end-users, actively pursue the insights of disabled persons, go to where they are, and bring them to where innovation takes place. Listen. Involve. Innovate. In order to do this comprehensively, inclusion cannot simply be on a voluntary basis; innovators must incorporate people with disabilities as paid consultants or employees who are compensated for the value of their insights. This is to everyone's benefit, from both humanitarian and economic points of view. It has been demonstrated that employers benefit financially from an inclusive workplace: inclusion can generate up to 28% higher revenue and 30% better performance on economic profit margin (Powers, 2017).

Inclusion in idea generation can and must be followed by inclusion in implementation. Historically speaking, people with disabilities have been left out of the research apparatus and thus marginalized from the kinds of trials that demonstrate effectiveness of technology. As technology develops, we must move toward true diverse participation in quality clinical trials, in which the promotion of broad involvement can pioneer healthcare and technological solutions that are truly relevant for disabled populations. Accessibility initiatives can advance science, and science can advance accessibility initiatives through the validation of valuable technologies that improve healthcare outcomes and patient well-being. While the case for increased diversity in clinical trials, which includes people with disabilities, is essentially self-evident, the practical logistics are far less so.

Clinical trial diversity that includes people with disabilities must begin with community engagement to identify and recruit participants, and it must be designed around technologies that are useful and usable for this population. It will be critical to measure outcomes that are relevant to the lives of these consumers. For instance, there are few objective measures of technological feasibility in *accessing* digital health technologies, which is critical in ensuring the usability of technology for people with disabilities (Klaassen et al., 2016). Tools used to measure the effectiveness of technologies used by people with disabilities should have objective standards with field usability testing, in which factors such as psychomotor skills are evaluated (de Joode et al., 2010; Kaufman et al., 2003). As objective measures for feasibility are increasingly used in the context of surmounting the challenges experienced by other underrepresented populations in research (e.g. low-income people and/or those who face language barriers), these standards should be applied for inclusion of those who have mobility challenges and other disabilities (Sarkar et al., 2016).

In addition to research on technology designed to benefit patients with disabilities, further studies should be conducted to evaluate clinician adoption of digital tools most likely to benefit the disabled community. Many metrics exist for evaluating clinician adoption of technology, the most notable being the Technology Acceptance Model (Charness & Boot, 2016). As gatekeepers of innovative therapies, clinicians must be included in digital study design. Usability studies are well established for technologies such as the electronic medical record (EMR), given that the Office of the National Coordinator for Health Information Technology requires that vendors test specific EMR capabilities with clinician end users and report their usability testing process. However, this usability standard is not yet established for healthcare applications (Rubin & Chisnell, 2008; Scott Kruse et al., 2017). This is particularly true for healthcare applications serving those with disabilities. Partnerships between disabled patients, physicians, vendors, and scientists can ensure a comprehensive approach to digital health research, eliciting value and adoption by both clinicians and patients.

Finally, the inclusion of people with disabilities is instrumental in the marketing of accessible technologies. Increasingly, health technology assessment (HTA) organizations have been involving the public and patients in their work, which was previously dominated by scientists, clinicians or industry (Sharma, 2019). It is possible that HTA can effectively include patient participation (Abelson et al., 2016). This inclusion could be monumental for persons with disabilities in meaningfully contributing to science, technological design, and their own health outcomes. This should be echoed. This should be amplified. People with disabilities should be visible, using technology, living their lives to their fullest capacity. Especially now, in this new era of medicine that intersects with technology, we should showcase the inclusion of people with disabilities so that their existence in our community is reflected by their presence in our culture. As a growing population, an important market force power and as valuable members of our society, people with disabilities represent the next frontier of comprehensive inclusion, and it is incumbent upon healthcare and technology to understand their needs and rise to this occasion.

The American Academy of Medical Colleges (AAMC) recently created a list of competencies for telehealth education to alleviate some of the lack in standardization. The guidelines are in six domains and include competencies for various levels of training, including physicians entering residency, recent graduates entering practice, and experienced faculty physicians (AAMC, 2021). Domain 2, Access and Equity in Telehealth, is relevant to addressing the needs of patients with disabilities using telehealth and is represented in the box below. The domain regarding access and equity in telehealth is intended to guide physician trainees to promote equitable access to care, by understanding telehealth delivery that addresses and mitigates cultural biases as well as physician bias for or against telehealth and that accounts for physical and mental disabilities and non-health-related individual and community needs and limitations (AAMC, 2021).

AAMC Telehealth Competencies Domain II: Access and Equity in Telehealth

Entering residency	Entering practice (recent residency graduate)	Experienced faculty physician (3–5 years post-residency)
1a. Describes one's own implicit and explicit biases and their implications when considering telehealth	1b. Describes and mitigates one's own implicit and explicit biases during telehealth encounters	1c. Role models and teaches how to recognize and mitigate biases during telehealth encounters
2a. Defines how telehealth can affect health equity and mitigate or amplify gaps in access to care	2b. Leverages technology to promote health equity and mitigate gaps in access to care	2c. Promotes and advocates the use of telehealth to promote health equity and access to care and to advocate for policy change in telehealth to reduce inequities
3a. When considering telehealth, assesses the patient's needs, preferences, access to, and potential cultural, social, physical, cognitive, and linguistic and other communication barriers to technology use	3b. When considering telehealth, accommodates the patient's needs, preferences, and potential cultural, social, physical, cognitive, and linguistic and communication barriers to technology use	3c. When considering telehealth, role models how to advocate for improved access to it and accommodates the patient's needs, preferences, and potential cultural, social, physical, cognitive, and linguistic and communication barriers to technology use

AAMC. (2021). *Telehealth competencies across the learning continuum.* AAMC New and Emerging Areas in Medicine Series. Washington, DC: AAMC.

KEY POINTS

Telehealth is a mechanism by which to bridge barriers that can impede access to healthcare.

People with disabilities have largely been underexplored as a public health group experiencing health disparities.

People with disabilities face particular healthcare challenges that can either be improved or exacerbated by advancements of telehealth.

Many behavioral health risks disproportionately affect the lives of people with disabilities.

Advancements in telehealth are particularly well suited for the management of chronic healthcare conditions that people with disabilities experience.

People with disabilities are increasingly reliant on electronic devices to improve their ability to interact with their environment.

In order for community-dwelling people with disabilities to live at home in a fully participatory way, technology must be developed that provides them with ways to interact with their environments.

Especially for people with disabilities, technology has the potential to provide an existence with reduced adverse health outcomes, reduced care coordination needs, and a reduced risk of long-term hospitalization.

As telehealth technologies are developed, the participation of people with disabilities in innovation must be paramount.

Inclusion in innovation must begin at the idea-generation phase and then be carried through to every other phase of technological development.

It is important to isolate and identify end users, actively pursue the insights of disabled persons, go to where they live, and bring them to where innovation is taking place.

CRITICAL THINKING EXCERCISES

1. Essentially by definition, disability creates deficits in people's ability to fully participate in parts of social life. How can technology be used to address some of the disparities that people with disabilities face? Describe one scenario in which technology has been used to address deficits caused by disability.

2. While some technology is accessible to many people, including those with disabilities, many more technological advancements are not designed with disability inclusion in mind. How can we incentivize and promote inclusion of people with disabilities in innovation?

3. Discuss the ways in which telehealth has been a benefit to the lives of people with disabilities. Discuss the ways in which telehealth might be detrimental to the lives of people with disabilities. How can we enhance benefits and reduce detriments?

REFERENCES

AAMC. (2021). *Telehealth competencies across the learning continuum. AAMC New and Emerging Areas in Medicine Series.* Washington, DC: AAMC.

Abelson, J., Wagner, F., DeJean, D., et al. (2016). Public and patient involvement in health technology assessment: A framework for action. *International Journal of Technology Assessment in Health Care, 32*(4), 256–264. https://doi.org/10.1017/S0266462316000362.

Anderson, M., & Perrin, A. (2021). *Disabled Americans are less likely to use technology.* Pew Research Center. Retrieved from: https://www.pewresearch.org/fact-tank/2017/04/07/disabled-americans-are-less-likely-to-use-technology/.

Baldassin, V., Shimizu, H. E., & Fachin-Martins, E. (2018). Computer assistive technology and associations with quality of life for individuals with spinal cord injury: A systematic review. *Quality of Life Research: An International Journal of Quality of Life Aspects of Treatment, Care and Rehabilitation, 27*(3), 597–607. https://doi.org/10.1007/s11136-018-1804-9.

Brodey, D. (2019). *1 billion disabled people just hit the business radar.* Forbes. www.forbes.com/sites/denisebrodey/2019/06/03/one-billion-disabled-people-just-hit-the-business-radar/?sh=309cf5814f27. [Accessed 1 November 2021].

Caggioni, L. (2019). *Project DIVA: Making the Google assistant more accessible.* https://experiments.withgoogle.com/project-diva. [Accessed 1 November 2021].

Carayon, P., Schoofs Hundt, A., Karsh, B.-T., et al. (2006). Work system design for patient safety: The SEIPS model. *Quality and Safety in Health Care, 15*(1), i50–i58. https://doi.org/10.1136/qshc.2005.015842.

Center for Medicare and Medicaid Services. (2018). *Information on Medicare telehealth.* Retrieved from: https://www.cms.gov/About-CMS/Agency-Information/OMH/Downloads/Information-on-Medicare-Telehealth-Report.pdf.

Centers for Disease Control. (2013). *CDC health disparities and inequalities report.* https://www.cdc.gov/minorityhealth/CHDIReport.html#anchor_1607954179.

Centers for Disease Control. (2020). *CDC in action: Preparing communities for potential spread of COVID-19.* https://stacks.cdc.gov/view/cdc/85304.

Centre for Excellence. (2020). In universal design. In *What is universal design?* http://universaldesign.ie/What-is-Universal-Design/. [Accessed 1 November 2021].

Chaet, D., Clearfield, R., Sabin, J. E., et al. (2017). Ethical practice in telehealth and telemedicine. *Journal of General Internal*

Medicine, 32(10), 1136–1140. https://doi.org/10.1007/s11606-017-4082-2.

Charness, N., & Boot, W. R. (2016). Chapter 20 —Technology, gaming, and social networking. In K. W. Schaie, & S. L. Willis (Eds.), *Handbook of the psychology of aging* (8th ed.). www.sciencedirect.com/topics/social-sciences/technology-acceptance-model. [Accessed 1 November 2021].

Chen, W.-L., Liou, A.-H. A., Chen, S.-C., et al. (2007). A novel home appliance control system for people with disabilities. *Disability and Rehabilitation: Assistive Technology, 2*(4), 201–206. https://doi.org/10.1080/17483100701456012.

Choney, S. (2019). *Microsoft's AI for accessibility grant winners: "You want to be seen as the person you are.* https://news.microsoft.com/features/microsofts-ai-for-accessibility-grant-winners-you-want-to-be-seen-as-the-person-you-are/. [Accessed 1 November 2021].

Davis, F. D., Bagozzi, R. P., & Warshaw, P. R. (1989). User acceptance of computer technology: A comparison of two theoretical models. *Management Science, 35*(8), 982–1003. http://www.jstor.org/stable/2632151.

de Joode, E., van Heugten, C., Verhey, F., et al. (2010). Efficacy and usability of assistive technology for patients with cognitive deficits: A systematic review. *Clinical Rehabilitation, 24*(8), 701–714. https://doi.org/10.1177/0269215510367551.

Donovan, R. (2016). *Return on disability.* www.rod-group.com. [Accessed 1 November 2021].

Emanuel, J. (2020). *Project Euphonia's personalized speech recognition for non-standard.* https://ai.googleblog.com/2019/08/project-euphonias-personalized-speech.html. [Accessed 1 November 2021].

Folan, A., Barclay, L., Cooper, C., et al. (2015). Exploring the experience of clients with tetraplegia utilizing assistive technology for computer access. *Disability and Rehabilitation: Assistive Technology, 10*(1), 46–52. https://doi.org/10.3109/17483107.2013.836686.

Holden, R. J., Carayon, P., Gurses, A. P., et al. (2013). Seips 2.0: A human factors framework for studying and improving the work of healthcare professionals and patients. *Ergonomics, 56*(11), 1669–1686. https://doi.org/10.1080/00140139.2013.838643.

Jones, M., Grogg, K., Anschutz, J., et al. (2008). A sip-and-puff wireless remote control for the Apple iPod. *Assistive Technology: The Official Journal of RESNA, 20*(2), 107–110. https://doi.org/10.1080/10400435.2008.10131937.

Kaufman, D. R., Patel, V. L., Hilliman, C., et al. (2003). Usability in the real world: Assessing medical information technologies in patients' homes. *Journal of Biomedical Informatics, 36*(1–2), 45–60. https://doi.org/10.1016/s1532-0464(03)00056-x.

Keramat, & Syed A., et al. (2021). Obesity, disability and self-perceived health outcomes in Australian adults: a longitudinal analysis using 14 annual waves of the HILDA cohort. *ClinicoEconomics and Outcomes Research.* 13. Gale Academic OneFile. link.gale.com/apps/doc/A679286097/AONE?u=sunysb&sid=bookmark-AONE&xid=79e861e6. [Accessed 30 September 2021].

Klaassen, B., van Beijnum, B. J. F., & Hermens, H. J. (2016). Usability in telemedicine systems – a literature survey.

International Journal of Medical Informatics, 93, 57–69. https://doi.org/10.1016/j.ijmedinf.2016.06.004.

Krahn, G. L., Walker, D. K., & Correa-De-Araujo, R. (2015). Persons with disabilities as an unrecognized health disparity population. *American Journal of Public Health, 105*(2), S198–S206. https://doi.org/10.2105/AJPH.2014.302182.

Noel, K., & Ellison, B. (2020). Inclusive innovation: 30 years after the ADA, how digital health innovation can promote accessibility for the next 30 years to come. *NPJ Digital Medicine, 3*(1), 1–3.

Powers, T. (2017). *Creating inclusive workplaces is a business imperative.* IBM. www.ibm.com/blogs/age-and-ability/2017/06/19/creating-inclusive-workplaces-business-imperative/. [Accessed 1 November 2021].

Riemer-Reiss, M. L., & Wacker, R. R. (2000). Factors associated with assistive technology discontinuance among individuals with disabilities. *Journal of Rehabilitation, 66*(3), 44–50.

Rigby, P., Ryan, S. E., & Campbell, K. A. (2011). Electronic aids to daily living and quality of life for persons with tetraplegia. *Disability and Rehabilitation: Assistive Technology, 6*(3), 260–267. https://doi.org/10.3109/17483107.2010.522678.

Rubin, J., & Chisnell, D. (2008). *Handbook of usability testing: How to plan, design, and conduct effective tests.* Wiley publishing, Inc. Indianapolis, Illinois. US.

Sarkar, U., Gourley, G. I., Lyles, C. R., et al. (2016). Usability of commercially available mobile applications for diverse patients. *Journal of General Internal Medicine, 31*(12), 1417–1426. https://doi.org/10.1007/s11606-016-3771-6.

SCI-Info (n.d.). *Spinal cord injury facts and statistics.* Quadriplegic, paraplegic and caregiver resource. www.sci-info-pages.com/facts.html. [Accessed 1 November 2021].

Scott Kruse, C., Krowski, N., Rodriguez, B., et al. (2017). Telehealth and patient satisfaction: A systematic review and narrative analysis. *BMJ Open, 7*(8), e016242. https://doi.org/10.1136/bmjopen-2017-016242.

Sharma, K. (2019). *Growing patient involvement in health technology assessment (HTA).* Decision Resources Group. https://decisionresourcesgroup.com/blog/growing-patient-involvement-health-technology-assessment-hta/. [Accessed 1 November 2021].

Venkatesh, V., & Davis, F. D. (2000). A theoretical extension of the technology acceptance model: Four longitudinal field studies. *Management Science, 46*(2), 186–204.

Woods, T. (2019). *"Age-Tech": The next frontier market for technology disruption.* www.forbes.com/sites/tinawoods/2019/02/01/age-tech-the-next-frontier-market-for-technology-disruption/#1406ea9d6c84. [Accessed 1 November 2021].

World Health Organization. (2011). *World report on disability.* www.who.int/publications/i/item/9789241564182. [Accessed 1 November 2021].

Young, D. & Edwards, E. (2020). Telehealth and disability: challenges and opportunities for care. National Health Law Program. https://healthlaw.org/telehealth-and-disability-challenges-and-opportunities-for-care/.

Educating Future Clinicians

11

Introducing Students to Telehealth: Creating Clinical Scenarios and Simulations for Interprofessional Training

Erin Hulfish, MD, FAAP

OBJECTIVES

1. Describe the essential components for preparing providers for telemedicine.
2. Describe the importance of communication as part of a virtual team.
3. Describe the process of building clinical interprofessional telesimulation scenarios.
4. Understand successful ways to implement an interprofessional simulation curriculum.

CHAPTER OUTLINE

KEY TERMS

Interprofessional team the members of the health care team that vary based on the patient and are of different primary disciplines

Simulation imitation of a situation or process

Telehealth the use of electronic information and communication technology to deliver health care services

Telesimulation the practice of telehealth in a simulated environment

Webside manner how to conduct yourself in a profession manner virtually

INTRODUCTION

Education in the art of telemedicine is rapidly becoming an important topic of consideration in many different ways. This education is needed for all levels of learners and extends beyond just the practicing physicians to include the entire clinical team. This chapter will focus on the immersive simulation experience of the interprofessional healthcare team. Topics will include who the team members are, how to build the clinical scenarios, the importance of tele-presence, and the ways to successfully integrate a telesimulation curriculum.

Simulation-based medical education has been a mainstay of teaching for many years. Not only does it allow healthcare students to practice all aspects of patient encounters in a safe and nonthreatening environment, but the experience can be replicated and repeated as necessary (Issenberg et al., 2005; Motola et al., 2013). Importantly, the cases can be adapted to a variety of healthcare professions and provide a mix of didactic and immersive simulated experiences (Kolb, 2001). Interprofessional education (IPE) including simulations has continued to be integrated in many different schools and has been shown to improve clinical care (Costello et al., 2017; Murphy, 2015; Riley et al., 2011; Zwarenstein et al., 2009).

The COVID-19 pandemic generated an imminent need for virtual telehealth visits in both the inpatient and the outpatient settings. There has been more emphasis now placed on the role of the interprofessional healthcare team in coordinating home care and continued health maintenance for high-quality patient care. Education now must be centered on how to work as a clinical interprofessional team in a virtual environment. The implementation of a telesimulation IPE curriculum will help fulfill educational gaps and teach learners to work effectively in a new virtual environment (Bond et al., 2019; Hilty et al., 2017).

PREPARING PROVIDERS FOR TELEMEDICINE

There are many differences in how providers need to communicate in a virtual environment, not only with their patients but within an interprofessional team. One of the biggest challenges to overcome is how to establish rapport and ensure trustworthiness. Some providers are naturally comfortable interacting with patients in a virtual environment and having themselves be viewed on camera; however, there are many who have difficulty with their virtual presence or interacting and establishing connection with the patient and/or team members. A first impression matters, and healthcare professionals who are not prepared to utilize telehealth could jeopardize the clinician-patient relationship, which could potentially lead to suboptimal healthcare delivery and overall lack of trust in the healthcare team (Agha et al., 2009). By utilizing and maximizing interactive training modules focusing on effective virtual communication techniques, one can have the same confidence in leading a telehealth visit and develop skills to foster the same high level of rapport in the virtual world as was previously achievable in a physical space. (Fraser, 2020; Keller & Carroll, 1994)

Webside Manner

Throughout their education, healthcare professionals are taught the importance of bedside manner, and how to effectively interact with patients to improve their outcomes and strengthen the patient-provider relationship. The same principles remain when moving to the virtual space and interacting with patients and other providers; this has been termed "webside" manner. Practicing some of the major components of webside manner in a simulated environment will allow better preparedness for actual clinical encounters (Sohn, 2020; Stephenson-Famy et al., 2015). Table 11.1 demonstrates the elements of good webside manner; items in bold are key for establishing rapport and engaging the patient.

Establishing Rapport

Establishing a connection is one of the core components of the clinician-patient relationship; while forming that connection in a virtual environment is challenging, it is essential for having an effective, fruitful visit and establishing follow-up care (Windover, 2014). Engaging the patient in "small talk" to ease into the visit will allow them to be put at ease and they will be more apt to respond better to questions. It is important to obtain background information about the patient, including prereading the chart or attending a preplanning meeting with the interprofessional team to understand all the patient concerns. The healthcare members on the telehealth visit should be properly introduced in a welcoming and friendly manner, and their roles explained to the patient. The telehealth environment is new to many, so giving time to explain how the visit will work, which may include looking at the electronic medical record (EMR) and assuring the patient of their privacy during the visit, will strengthen the relationship.

During the visit, providers will need to demonstrate active listening to validate the patient's concerns and points of view. Utilization of active listening techniques will also keep providers more engaged in the conversation (Morony et al., 2018). Excessive movement of the body during the interview can be distracting. Avoiding this is especially difficult for those who are used to expressing themselves with more body language during a visit; however, appropriate and timely use of hand gestures, such as a "thumbs-up" sign or a wave, can communicate to the patient and others that the message is being understood and that the interview is progressing well. It is important to also establish empathy during a video visit. Techniques such as leaning forward toward the camera and nodding, as well as stating out loud the emotions felt, provide support for patients during the telehealth session. Domain 3 of the AAMC telehealth competencies refers to communication and may be helpful to review here.

Effective Communication Strategies

Different skill sets are necessary depending on who is involved in the communication exchange. Communication exchanges between two healthcare professionals are different from those taking place between a healthcare professional and their patient. The AAMC has recently published a set of competencies for telehealth (see Table 11.1) and there have been existing telehealth competencies from the American Nursing Association including assessment of communication via telehealth (AAMC, 2021; ANA, 1999;

TABLE 11.1	Techniques for Good Webside Manner
Camera Angle	Place camera at or above eye level Provider should be positioned in the middle of the frame
Eye contact	Look at the camera during the interview to establish good "eye contact" Consider rotating the screen back to maintain eye contact and still have good visualization of the computer screen
Microphone usage	Be aware of any adventitious noises (e.g., pen clicking, foot tapping) that may be distracting During interprofessional meetings, mute microphone when not speaking
Appearance	Dress professionally Accentuate emotions; nod and smile
Environmental factors	Ensure privacy during interview No food or drinks during interview
Lighting	Face should be well lit on screen Light coming in from behind participants will cast shadows on face

Source: Barfield et al., 1995; McCulloch, 1999; Williams et al., 2015; Colleges, 2020a.

AAMC Telehealth Competencies Domain 3: Communication via Telehealth

Entering residency	Entering practice (recent residency graduate)	Experienced faculty physician (3–5 years post-residency)
1a. Develops an effective rapport with patients via real or simulated video visits, attending to eye contact, tone, body language, and nonverbal cues	1b. Develops an effective rapport with patients via video visits, attending to eye contact, tone, body language, and nonverbal cues	1c. Role models and teaches effective rapport-building with patients via video visits, attending to eye contact, tone, body language, and nonverbal cues
2a. Assesses the environment during real or simulated video visits, including attending to disruptions related to privacy, lighting, sound, and attire	2b. Establishes therapeutic relationships and environments during video visits, including attending to disruptions related to privacy, lighting, sound, and attire	2c. Role models effective therapeutic relationships and environments
3a. Explains how remote patients' social supports and healthcare providers can be incorporated into telehealth interactions and the care plan (e.g., asynchronous communication and the storage and forwarding of data)	3b. Determines situations in which patients' social supports and healthcare providers should be incorporated into telehealth interactions, with the patients' consent, to provide optimal care	3c. Role models and teaches how to incorporate patients' social supports into telehealth interactions, with the patients' consent, to provide optimal care

AAMC. (2021). *Telehealth competencies across the learning continuum.* AAMC New and Emerging Areas in Medicine Series. Washington, DC: AAMC.

Colleges, 2020b). With the rise of telehealth utilization among all disciplines, there may be further competency developments as well as interprofessional telehealth competency development as for in-person teams (Bridges et al., 2011; Consortium, 2016; Frank et al., 2010; Weller, 2015).

During Provider-to-Patient Encounters

Creating effective communication is key in delivering high-quality healthcare (Iversen et al., 2020). A telemedicine visit should be conducted in much the same format as a traditional in-office visit. The most important aspect is the initial welcoming and introduction to the technology and the structure of the visit. The healthcare professional would benefit from establishing rapport so that the patient is comfortable in the environment and feels able to ask any questions pertaining to their healthcare. The healthcare professional may choose to engage the patient in conversation about their health and refer to any previous visits. It is important to avoid any medical jargon and be cognizant of the patient's cultural and linguisitic background (Agha et al., 2009; Duran & Popescu, 2014; Gustin et al., 2020; Morony et al., 2018).

The healthcare professional may consider creating an agenda for the visit incorporating any concerns that the patient has, and may enlist their help in creating a focused visit. Open-ended questions should be utilized while taking a background history with a patient, allowing the patient to share their health story. The healthcare professional should incorporate active listening skills to engage with the patient. When building a plan, it is essential to have the patient participate to know what can be accomplished. By utilizing techniques such as teach-back (Morony et al., 2018), the provider will be able to assess the patient's understanding and decide upon steps to move forward. Finally, the provider should establish a plan for follow-up and where this will take place (either in person or with telehealth). A summary of how to structure a telehealth patient visit is given in Table 11.2.

COMMUNICATION IN AN INTERPROFESSIONAL TEAM

Interprofessional communication works in much the same way as patient and provider visits. Establish an open and friendly environment that is built on collaboration. Ensure that roles are defined and respected during the encounter and that everyone shares equally in responsibility (Gustin et al., 2020; Kurtz, 2005; Weller, 2015). Team members must:

- promote contributions from and recognize the efforts of all involved;
- remain dynamic and open to modifying individual duties based on need;

TABLE 11.2	Summary of Patient Visit
Introduction to the session	Introduce the technology and ensure privacy to visit Engage in small talk Refer to any previous sessions' topics Avoid medical jargon Elicit any culture-specific concerns
Goal-oriented visit	Elicit concerns that the patient has Establish agenda and focus for the visit collaboratively
Elicit a history	Use open-ended questions Employ active listening
Patient participation in plan building	Have patient participate in building a plan Check for understanding using teach-back techniques
Close and follow-up	Establish plan for follow-up

- set goals collaboratively and operationalize them in ways that can be easily measured;
- agree on the communication channel and the frequency of communication.

INCORPORATION OF INTERPROFESSIONAL TELESIMULATION ACTIVITIES

Experiential learning theories use simulation to teach and solidify concepts in interprofessional teamwork and communication. Despite its proven utility, creating a telehealth simulation curriculum remains a challenging endeavor. Though creating an immersive and comprehensive telesimulation program is challenging, when added to the curriculum it will enhance learning, solidify concepts, and improve overall satisfaction with the course (Costello et al., 2017; Ericsson, 2008; Kolb, 2001; Motola et al., 2013; Taylor & Hamdy, 2013).

Champions

It is essential that there are selected champions for the disciplines who are invested in creating and teaching an interprofessional simulation course. These members do not have to have simulation experience. Having champions will help the recruitment not only of learners but of other facilitators in their respective fields to teach and work with the different course directors to find a way to implement the simulation sessions into the curriculum. Having a diverse team of champions will help to ensure that the aims of each course are achieved and that all learning objectives are incorporated.

Another essential part of the simulation champion team is the members of the simulation center itself. It is essential to engage the members of the simulation center early to get them involved in simulation creation. They will know what capabilities the center currently has in terms of technology and member participation. Also, in a time of pandemic and social distancing, the simulation center coordinators will have the information about what is allowable for the center. By providing a new virtual space to create and run interprofessional activities, this will provide the center with an outlet and facilitators to run educational cases, further endearing them to the IPE cause.

Creation of Simulation Cases

Start Small

When first building an interprofessional telehealth simulation curriculum, there can be a push to incorporate as many schools and learners as possible into the initial simulations. While this is always the goal of teaching—to reach as many students as possible—starting small with just two or three different interprofessional groups will help keep the initial simulations manageable.

Enlist the other interprofessional directors to form a small simulation-focused committee to develop cases with clear learning objectives that will be easily integrated into courses. This committee can also be publicized as an additional resource to other programs looking to integrate IPE activities into their schools to help with continued educational advancement. The case can be developed from real-life cases or from the adaptation of previous in-person IPE simulation cases. (Baker et al., 2008; Collins et al., 2019; Costello et al., 2017). Table 11.3 reviews examples of initial simulation cases, including the interprofessionals involved and topics to be explored.

Expansion

Creation of a core case list that encompasses a variety of patient conditions is a good starting point from which the cases can be adapted for a variety of different environments. Telehealth and interprofessional interactions do not occur in only one place; they can involve patients in either a hospital or another acute or subacute center, outpatient offices, emergency and urgent care centers, or home-based patients. Each situation brings a different set

TABLE 11.3	Examples of Initial Simulation Cases	
Case examples	**Interprofessionals involved**	**Initial case**
Discharge stroke patient from the hospital	MD (primary and subspecialty), RN, RT, PT, OT, SLP, SW, RD	• How to safely discharge from the hospital • What services and evaluations are needed for home? • What is the appropriate follow-up timeline?
Congestive heart failure patient at home	MD (primary and subspecialty), RN, SW, pharmacist	• Medication compliance and interactions • Remote patient monitoring tools (blood pressure, weight, O_2 saturations) • What support systems are in place?
Psychiatric patient: ED-to-inpatient transfer	MD (primary and subspecialty), RN, clerk, SW, registration, transport service	• How to call a consult? • Define the process for using telemedicine
New diagnosis diabetes hospital follow-up	MD, SW, RD, RN	• Medication compliance • Dietary compliance • Adjustments to home and social support

ED, Emergency department; *MD*, medical doctor; *OT*, occupational therapist; *PT*, physical therapist; *RD*, registered dietician; *RN*, registered nurse; *RT*, respiratory therapist; *SLP*, speech and language pathologist; *SW*, social worker.

of challenges and will allow for numerous expansions of base cases (Sharma et al., 2011).

The level of learner targeted can also be used to expand upon the scenarios created. Cases can be developed for undergraduate- and graduate-level education as well as for practicing clinicians. The complexity and variety of learners can be increased depending upon needs (Cameron et al., 2009; Riley et al., 2011; Walters et al., 2017). Again, by using published telehealth competencies in combination with the competencies of the Interprofessional Education Collaborative, a larger library of cases can be created and adapted for continued course development (Brashers et al., 2020; Colleges, 2020b; Hilty et al., 2017, 2018). Table 11.4 includes examples of how to expand upon interprofessional base cases to develop a more complex scenario.

Video Recording

One of the most important aspects of simulation is the feedback it provides for the learners, and this is especially important with telesimulations. Providers can be very anxious and preoccupied with how they appear on camera, and this can be seen in their interactions during telemedicine visits. By video recording telesimulations and having the learners practice and view their own recordings, they will be able to become more comfortable with themselves on camera and provide a smoother, more effective visit.

SUCCESSFUL WAYS OF INCORPORATING INTERPROFESSIONAL TELEHEALTH EDUCATION

So far, we have spoken to the importance of education, the creation of the curriculum, the do's and the don'ts for building telesimulations, and how to prepare providers for telemedicine by using telesimulations. In the next section, we will look at successful ways of implementing the new curriculum.

Enlist Stakeholders

Once a group of champions has been formed, it is essential that the deans and/or any other curriculum stakeholders be approached and invested into the simulation curriculum. There may already be small interprofessional activities within the different disciplines, and finding ways of integrating into those curricula can be essential in implementing the course. Stakeholders also want to ensure that there are more than just stand-alone simulations being offered and to see

TABLE 11.4 Examples of Expanded Interprofessional Cases

Case examples	Interprofessionals involved	Initial case	Expansion
Discharge stroke patient from the hospital	MD (primary and subspecialty), RN, RT, PT, OT, SLP, SW, RD	• How to safely discharge from the hospital • What services and evaluations are needed for home? • What is the appropriate follow-up timeline?	• Another potential neurologic event at home • How to evaluate • Who to call
Congestive heart failure patient at home	MD (primary and subspecialty), RN, SW, pharmacist	• Medication compliance and interactions • Remote patient monitoring tools (blood pressure, weight, O_2 saturations) • What support systems are in place	• Worsening congestive heart failure • Try medication adjustment • Increased RN visits • Add in additional IPs
New diagnosis diabetes, hospital follow-up	MD, SW, RD, RN	• Medication compliance • Dietary compliance • Adjustments to home and social support	• Difficulty coping with diagnosis and diet • Support groups • Additional IPs • Medication adjustment

IP, Interprofessional; *MD*, medical doctor; *OT*, occupational therapist; *PT*, physical therapist; *RD*, registered dietician; *RN*, registered nurse; *RT*, respiratory therapist; *SLP*, speech and language pathologist; *SW*, social worker.

where value can be added to their curriculum and potentially supplement other areas that the schools need; these can include interprofessional conferences, workshops, and interest groups (Boet et al., 2014; Potosky, 2014).

Being familiar with the different schools' accreditation requirements for interprofessional education is also very important. An increasing number of programs are including interprofessional education into their accreditation but lack the high-quality integrative and immersive programs to engage learners. Know which schools require interprofessional education for their learners and for their accreditation, and target those courses (Reeves, 2012). Once the course is established, it will be easier to add more professionals to the core class or divide the curriculum to reach a wider array of learners.

Manage Expectations

Even once the stakeholders are engaged, the champions are arranged, and the curriculum developed, there is still the next phase: implementation of the curriculum. This task is the most challenging so far, as the logistics of finding a time for all groups to meet that works within the year's curriculum are difficult. Do not be discouraged if the initial planning takes longer than expected. Be flexible with timing and engage the stakeholders to find a way to integrate the modules into the curriculum. One of the advantages of a telehealth simulation is that the learners can be at a variety of different sites, as can the facilitators (Collins et al., 2019). This leads to less conflict with traveling to distant sites and is more easily adapted for a variety of schedules.

The use of telehealth technologies can more easily allow for implementation in either a synchronous or an asynchronous fashion. In an asynchronous format, learners may watch modules either within their own classes or on their own followed by several synchronous simulations. Allow for the presence of facilitators from the different schools to help guide

discussions afterwards and ensure all learning perspectives are represented. The flexibility of telesimulations is also enhanced by the ease with which scenarios can be rapidly repeated without needing significant time to set up a room.

Choose a Telehealth Platform

Many institutions have adopted new telehealth platforms that contain passwords, and institutionally protected software. All members of the team should have access to the telehealth platform and should have been trained on how to use it appropriately. Many audiovisual conferencing platforms are now available; however, to maintain a level of realism, utilize a platform that the healthcare professionals will use when they interact with their actual patients (Pourmand et al., 2018). In this way the course can also offer real-time training on the same equipment that students will use in the field.

Depending on the resources available, using a simulation center (which may have access to either standardized patients or mannequins) to implement the interprofessional simulation scenarios can be beneficial (Sharma et al., 2011). If using the simulation center to facilitate the encounters, ensure that the virtual technological platform will also work with the center's computer system and security. It is important to rehearse the interprofessional simulations to ensure that the equipment is working properly for the providers.

CONCLUSION

Interprofessional education continues to be an important core pillar for clinician education and engagement. By developing a course that includes a combination of didactic (combination of both synchronous and asynchronous activities) and interactive telesimulations, clinicians will develop more confidence and experience in interacting with an interprofessional team and improving patient care through telehealth.

REVIEW QUESTIONS

1. What are three elements of effective communication strategies?
2. What are strategies for telesimulation incorporation into a curriculum?

? CRITICAL THINKING EXERCISES

Using the case tables in this chapter as a guide, create a clinical interprofessional scenario. Consider the professionals who could be involved and indicate their roles for the case. Consider how this could be implemented at your institution, and what the supports and barriers would be to the implementation.

For the final exercise, implement the above scenario in a simulated environment. Ensure that you record the encounter, and gather a small focus group to review the video. Assign group members a specific task for the review, such as webside manner, communication, or technology issues, to provide a specific focus for the review.

REFERENCES

AAMC (2021). *Telehealth competencies across the learning continuum. AAMC New and Emerging Areas in Medicine Series.* Washington, DC: AAMC.

Agha, Z., Schapira, R. M., Laud, P. W., et al. (2009). Patient satisfaction with physician-patient communication during telemedicine. *Telemedicine Journal and E-Health, 15*(9), 830–839. https://doi.org/10.1089/tmj.2009.0030.

American Nursing Association. (1999). *Competencies for telehealth technologies in nursing.* Washington, DC.

Baker, C., Pulling, C., McGraw, R., et al. (2008). Simulation in interprofessional education for patient-centred collaborative care. *Journal of Advanced Nursing, 64*(4), 372–379. https://doi.org/10.1111/j.1365-2648.2008.04798.x.

Barfield, W., Zeltzer, D., Sheridan, T., et al. (1995). Presence and performance within virtual environments. In *Virtual environments and advanced interface design* (pp. 473–513). USA: Oxford University Press.

Boet, S., Bould, M. D., Layat Burn, C., et al. (2014). Twelve tips for a successful interprofessional team-based high-fidelity simulation education session. *Medical Teacher, 36*(10), 853–857. https://doi.org/10.3109/0142159X.2014.923558.

Bond, W. F., Barker, L. T., Cooley, K. L., et al. (2019). A simple low-cost method to integrate telehealth interprofessional team members during in situ simulation. *Simulation in Healthcare: Journal of the Society for Simulation in Healthcare, 14*(2), 129–136. https://doi.org/10.1097/SIH.0000000000000357.

Brashers, V., Haizlip, J., & Owen, J. A. (2020). The ASPIRE Model: Grounding the IPEC core competencies for interprofessional collaborative practice within a foundational framework. *Journal of Interprofessional Care, 34*(1), 128–132. https://doi.org/10.1080/13561820.2019.1624513.

Bridges, D. R., Davidson, R. A., Odegard, P. S., et al. (2011). Interprofessional collaboration: Three best practice models of interprofessional education. *Medical Education Online, 16.* https://doi.org/10.3402/meo.v16i0.6035.

Cameron, A., Rennie, S., DiProspero, L., et al. (2009). An introduction to teamwork: Findings from an evaluation of an interprofessional education experience for 1000 first-year health science students. *Journal of Allied Health, 38*(4), 220–226.

Colleges, A. (2020a). *Conducting interviews during the coronavirus pandemic.*

Colleges, A. (2020b). *New and emerging areas in medicine series: Telehealth competencies.* https://www.aamc.org/what-we-do/mission-areas/medical-education/conducting-interviews-during-coronavirus-pandemic https://www.aamc.org/data-reports/report/telehealth-competencies.

Collins, C., Lovett, M., Biffar, D., et al. (2019). The use of remote and traditional faciliation to evaluate telesimulation to support interprofessional education and processing in healthcare simulation training. SpringSim 2019 [8732914] (2019 Spring Simulation Conference, SpringSim 2019). In *2019 Spring simulation conference.* Institute of Electrical and Electronics Engineers, Inc. https://doi.org/10.23919/SpringSim.2019.8732914.

Consotium, I. E. (2016). *IPEC core competencies for interprofessional collaborative practice. 2016 update.*

Costello, M., Huddleston, J., Atinaja-Faller, J., et al. (2017). Simulation as an effective strategy for interprofessional education. *Clinical Simulation in Nursing, 13*(12), 624–627. https://doi.org/10.1016/j.ecns.2017.07.008.

Duran, V., & Popescu, A.-D. (2014). The challenge of multicultural communication in virtual teams. *Procedia – Social and Behavioral Sciences, 109*, 365–369. https://doi.org/10.1016/j.sbspro.2013.12.473.

Ericsson, K. A. (2008). Deliberate practice and acquisition of expert performance: A general overview. *Academic Emergency Medicine: Official Journal of the Society for Academic Emergency Medicine, 15*(11), 988–994. https://doi.org/10.1111/j.1553-2712.2008.00227.x.

Frank, J. R., Snell, L. S., Cate, O. T., et al. (2010). Competency-based medical education: Theory to practice. *Medical Teacher, 32*(8), 638–645. https://doi.org/10.3109/0142159X.2010.501190.

Fraser Rebecca, L. (2020). *Prep for success in your virtual interview.* Association of American Medical Colleges.

Gustin, T. S., Kott, K., & Rutledge, C. (2020). Telehealth etiquette training: A guideline for preparing interprofessional teams for successful encounters. *Nurse Educator, 45*(2), 88–92. https://doi.org/10.1097/NNE.0000000000000680.

Hilty, D. M., Maheu, M. M., Drude, K. P., et al. (2018). The need to implement and evaluate telehealth competency frameworks to ensure quality care across behavioral health professions. *Academic Psychiatry: The Journal of the American Association of Directors of Psychiatric Residency Training and the Association for Academic Psychiatry, 42*(6), 818–824. https://doi.org/10.1007/s40596-018-0992-5.

Hilty, D., Maheu, M., Drude, K., et al. (2017). Telebehavioral health, telemental health, e-therapy and e-health competencies: The need for an interprofessional framework. *Journal of Technology in Behavioral Science, 2*, 1–19. https://doi.org/10.1007/s41347-017-0036-0.

Issenberg, S. B., McGaghie, W. C., Petrusa, E. R., et al. (2005). Features and uses of high-fidelity medical simulations that lead to effective learning: A BEME systematic review. *Medical Teacher, 27*(1), 10–28. https://doi.org/10.1080/01421590500046924.

Iversen, E. D., Wolderslund, M. O., Kofoed, P.-E., et al. (2020). Codebook for rating clinical communication skills based on the Calgary-Cambridge Guide. *BMC Medical Education, 20*(1), 140. https://doi.org/10.1186/s12909-020-02050-3.

Keller, V. F., & Carroll, J. G. (1994). A new model for physician-patient communication. *Patient Education and Counseling, 23*(2), 131–140. https://doi.org/10.1016/0738-3991(94)90051-5.

Kolb, D. A., Boyatzis, R. E., & Mainemelis, C. (2001). Experiential learning theory: Previous research and new directions. In *Perspectives on thinking, learning, and cognitive styles* (pp. 227–248). Routledge.

Kurtz, S. (2005). *Teaching and learning communication skills in medicine* (2nd ed.). Abingdon Oxon, UK: Radcliffe Medical Press.

McCulloch, M. S. (1999). Video conferencing systems: Telepresence and selection interviews. *Contemporary Ergonomics*, 133–137.

Morony, S., Weir, K., Duncan, G., et al. (2018). Enhancing communication skills for telehealth: Development and implementation of a teach-back intervention for a national maternal and child health helpline in Australia. *BMC Health Services Research*, *18*(1), 162. https://doi.org/10.1186/s12913-018-2956-6.

Motola, I., Devine, L. A., Chung, H. S., et al. (2013). Simulation in healthcare education: A best evidence practical guide. AMEE guide No. 82. *Medical Teacher*, *35*(10), e1511–e1530. https://doi.org/10.3109/0142159X.2013.818632.

Murphy, J. I., & Nimmagadda, J. (2015). Partnering to provide simulated learning to address Interprofessional Education Collaborative core competencies. *Journal of Interprofessional Care*, *29*(3), 258–259. https://doi.org/10.3109/13561820.2014.942779.

Potosky, D. (2014). Virtually experiential classrooms. In *Developments in business simulation and experiential learning: Proceedings of the annual ABSEL conference* (Vol. 29).

Pourmand, A., Lee, H., Fair, M., et al. (2018). Feasibility and usability of tele-interview for medical residency interview. *Western Journal of Emergency Medicine*, *19*(1), 80–86. https://doi.org/10.5811/westjem.2017.11.35167.

Reeves, S. (2012). The rise and rise of interprofessional competence. *Journal of Interprofessional Care*, *26*, 253–255. https://doi.org/10.3109/13561820.2012.695542.

Riley, W., Davis, S., Miller, K., et al. (2011). Didactic and simulation nontechnical skills team training to improve perinatal patient outcomes in a community hospital. *Joint Commission Journal on Quality and Patient Safety*, *37*(8), 357–364. https://doi.org/10.1016/s1553-7250(11)37046-8.

Sharma, S., Boet, S., Kitto, S., et al. (2011). Interprofessional simulated learning: The need for "sociological

fidelity". *Journal of Interprofessional Care*, *25*, 81–83. https://doi.org/10.3109/13561820.2011.556514.

Sohn, E. (2020). *"Residency, med school interviews go virtual: What to know"*. Medscape Medical News. https://www.medscape.com/viewarticle/932803.

Stephenson-Famy, A., Houmard, B. S., Oberoi, S., et al. (2015). Use of the interview in resident candidate selection: A review of the literature. *Journal of Graduate Medical Education*, *7*(4), 539–548. https://doi.org/10.4300/JGME-D-14-00236.1.

Taylor, D. C. M., & Hamdy, H. (2013). Adult learning theories: Implications for learning and teaching in medical education: AMEE guide No. 83. *Medical Teacher*, *35*(11), e1561–e1572. https://doi.org/10.3109/0142159X.2013.828153.

Walters, B., Potetz, J., & Fedesco, H. N. (2017). Simulations in the classroom: An innovative active learning experience. *Clinical Simulation in Nursing*, *13*(12), 609–615.

Weller, J. (2015). *Assessing teamwork and communication in the health professions*. Society of Critical Care Medicine. http://www.sccm.org/Communications/Critical-Connections/Archives/Pages/Assessing-Teamwork-and-Communication-in-the-Health-Professions.aspx.

Williams, K., Kling, J. M., Labonte, H. R., et al. (2015). Videoconference interviewing: Tips for success. *Journal of Graduate Medical Education*, *7*(3), 331–333. https://doi.org/10.4300/JGME-D-14-00507.1.

Windover, A.K., Boissy, A., Rice, T.W., et al. (2014). The REDE model of healthcare communication: optimizing relationship as a therapeutic agent. *J Patient Exper.* 1. 8–13.

Zwarenstein, M., Goldman, J., & Reeves, S. (2009). Interprofessional collaboration: Effects of practice-based interventions on professional practice and healthcare outcomes. *Cochrane Database of Systematic Reviews*, *3*. https://doi.org/10.1002/14651858.CD000072.pub2. CD000072.

12

In-Depth Remote Physical Assessment: The Musculoskeletal Exam

Charles M. Fisher, PT, MPT, MBA and JeMe Cioppa-Mosca, PT, MBA

"Providing high quality telehealth care is both an art and a science"

HSS Physical Therapist

OBJECTIVES

1. Assesses the environment during video visits, attending to attire, disruptions, privacy, lighting, sound, etc. for physical assessment.
2. Explains equipment required for conducting physical assessment via telehealth.
3. Explains limitations of and minimum requirements for local equipment, including common patient-owned devices.
4. Conducts an appropriate physical examination or collects relevant data on clinical status during a telehealth encounter, including guiding the patient or tele-presenter.
5. Describes when patient safety is at risk, including when and how to escalate care (e.g. converts to in-person visit or emergency response) during a telehealth physical exam assessment.
6. Demonstrates interprofessional teamwork in assessment of physical virtual assessment.

CHAPTER OUTLINE

KEY TERMS

Goniometer protractor-like tool for measuring joint range of motion

Manual muscle test (MMT) method of assessing objective strength of a muscle

Range of motion (ROM) movement of a joint from end point to end point

Red flag warning sign prior to providing care

Special test specific advanced diagnostic test, per body region or nature of complaint, to assist in confirming a diagnosis or with differential diagnosis

Tele-provider clinician who provides care through medium of telehealth

INTRODUCTION TO TELEHEALTH EXAMINATION AND CARE

Conducting a physical assessment through telehealth is not synonymous with providing an in-person assessment. A thorough telehealth physical assessment requires a different set of skills—a clinician's use of strong subjective questioning, clear communication, a sound understanding of functional movement patterns—and a systematic process that can differentially diagnose, treat, or refer as needed. It is challenging to conduct a thorough and objective telehealth evaluation due to the inability to perform hands-on assessment, provide tactile cues, and observe patient movement patterns in three dimensions.

This chapter will provide education and guidance on conducting a competent telehealth physical assessment of the musculoskeletal patient, regardless of specialty. In-depth follow-up may be indicated based on the results of the examination.

CONSIDERATIONS FOR TELEHEALTH PHYSICAL ASSESSMENT SESSION SETUP

An in-person physical examination is typically done in an appropriate clinical setting that contains the necessary supplies and equipment to optimize the clinician's ability to best examine the patient and achieve the goals of the examination. There is an examination table to allow the examination of patients in positions other than standing, robes for patients to allow observation of necessary body regions, and there are tape measures, goniometers, and scales to allow objective testing and measurement. There is appropriate lighting in the exam room which allows the provider to observe the patient with ease. The provider is able to move around the room to examine the patient from various perspectives to visualize the patient in the three different planes of motion: the sagittal, frontal, and transverse planes.

In a telehealth physical examination, it is important to account for any and all variables from both the patient and provider perspectives that are not typically present in an in-person clinical setting. This will help to ensure the examination can be completed in an accurate and thorough manner. Having the patient or tele-provider leave the screen to retrieve an item disrupts the flow of the examination and is inefficient.

Patient

Patients being evaluated through telehealth are encouraged to go online to become familiar with the logging-on process, as well as to complete any preexamination requirements prior to the scheduled appointment. For the

TABLE 12.1 General Clothing Recommendations	
Body region	**Recommendation**
Lumbar/thoracic spine	Men may remove shirt; women may use a tank top
Lower extremity	Wear shorts and remove shoes and socks
Cervical spine/shoulder	Men may remove shirt; women may use a tank top
Elbow/wrist/hand	Wear a shirt with short or no sleeves

Source: HSS Rehabilitation Telehealth Evaluation Guidelines for Musculoskeletal Physical Therapy.

evaluation, they should log in early to ensure there are no connectivity problems which would result in delays and limit the time the tele-provider has available to complete the examination.

Patients should be dressed in appropriate clothing to allow the tele-provider to observe the area of concern. Of note, it is sometimes indicated to examine body regions other than the area of concern to assess for contributing factors (e.g., looking at foot arches for knee, hip or back pain) as well as appropriate clothing allows, or the tele-provider may need to observe for items such as edema and ecchymosis or evaluate the status of incisions and wounds. Appropriate clothing also allows for observation of posture and functional movement of the area of concern. For general patient clothing recommendations, see Table 12.1.

Lighting is one crucial aspect of telehealth care that is not a factor with in-person care. Poor or misplaced lighting can inhibit a tele-provider's ability to capitalize on the observation portion of the physical exam. Lighting setups for telehealth may utilize different sources of light, such as indoor lighting, lamps, or natural sunlight. The most important principle is to have the light source in front of the patient. Avoid having the camera face the window or other light source, as that would result in a dark and shadowy image.

With the patient wearing the appropriate clothing, and the light source in an ideal position, the camera setup is vitally important to allow tele-providers to observe the patient in various scenarios. A portion of the exam may require close-up camera shots for examinations such as looking an incision, while other parts of the exam may need to see a whole-body motion such as squatting or touching the toes. The "camera considerations" section later will provide both general and detailed instructions on how to optimize camera setup and usage.

In a telehealth setting, the equipment and space for an examination are considerations that are not needed in a live setting. The space in which the patient will be examined should correlate with the examination focus. Examination of the elbow, wrist, and hand may be conducted using a smaller area with a tabletop to assist in supporting the upper extremity for examination. Examination of the shoulders may necessitate lying supine with arms raised overhead; patients may need to lie reversed in bed to allow for this movement to avoid their arms hitting the headboard. Regardless of the body part under consideration, space may be needed to allow for both small motions and full body movements in the same examination. Without

the appropriate space, the camera would not be able to capture them for the tele-provider to observe effectively.

Given that some objective testing, such as strength testing, is limited through telehealth, having patients use household objects (Table 12.2) or equipment sent to them in advance, such as resistance bands (Table 12.3), will assist in providing a level of objective assessment. Having any items present which may or will be used in the examination will help to make the examination more efficient and contiguous.

Tele-provider

All the considerations of telehealth assessment for the patient can be applied to the tele-provider. Tele-providers should perform the necessary training and due diligence to conduct telehealth sessions prior to live telehealth patient care. This includes being familiar with the software which the visits will occur within and common troubleshooting measures to assist when issues arise. Tele-providers should also understand considerations for objective testing given that this ability is limited in telehealth care (Box 12.1).

As the patient should be dressed in appropriate clothing, the tele-provider should present professionally as if the examination were in person. If the tele-provider is conducting the examination from their home or office, it important to have a professional background. Avoid personal artifacts and clutter, and keep in mind that you may need to move the camera as part of the examination process, which will show more of the area you are in.

The light source should be in front of the tele-provider to allow the patient to fully see the provider for the duration of the examination. To facilitate easier communication and limit background distractions, it is recommended that the tele-provider perform the examination in a private space.

TABLE 12.2   Resistance From Household Items

Item	Approximate weight (lb)
Bottle of water (450 mL or 16 oz); wine bottle	1
Quart of milk (950 mL); 1-L bottle of soda	1
Half-gallon of milk (1.9 L); 2-L soda bottle (full); unopened bottle of wine (750 mL)	4–5
Gallon of milk (3.8 L)	8

Source: HSS Rehabilitation Telehealth Evaluation Guidelines for Musculoskeletal Physical Therapy.

TABLE 12.3   Resistance From Resistance Bands

Color	Approximate resistance at 100% elongation in lb
Yellow	3
Red	3.7
Green	4.6
Blue	5.8
Black	7.3

Source: Theraband website https://www.theraband.com/theraband-professional-non-latex-resistance-bands-25-yard-roll.html. Accessed 11/28/20

BOX 12.1

- Objective testing considerations for musculoskeletal telehealth examination
- For specific joint ROM, use a goniometer against the computer screen.
- Use literature-based ROM values for functional movement testing.
- Functional testing is preferred to specific strength testing—consider patient's goals.
- For specific strength testing, if full ROM against gravity, MMT grade is at least 3/5.
  - Patient can perform self over-pressure to grade > 3/5.
- Have the patient perform self-palpation if appropriate.
- For special testing, consider ways patient can self-perform.
- Simple qualifiers (painful/pain-free, restricted/not restricted) can be valid and reliable.

MMT, Manual muscle test; *ROM*, range of movement.
Source: HSS Rehabilitation Telehealth Evaluation Guidelines for Musculoskeletal Physical Therapy.

If a private space is not an option, earphones and a microphone are both needed to communicate effectively with the patient and, most importantly, to maintain their privacy. Earphones and microphones reduce background noise and allow for clearer communication. Wireless microphones and earphones allow for continued communication when demonstrating movements away from the computer.

Any equipment needs for the examination should be readily accessible to the tele-provider during the examination. These are body region–specific and may include a model of a particular joint for patient education, a goniometer to measure **range of motion (ROM)** on the computer screen, or a prop such as a cane to examine or explain an exercise.

Camera Setup and Considerations

Optimizing camera setup is important for the tele-provider to successfully observe the area being examined. General camera concepts to achieve this are to tilt the laptop down if propped up (Fig. 12.1), hold the phone for close-up (Fig. 12.2), flip the phone horizontally to capture the entire body (Fig. 12.3), and lower the camera/laptop and position closely to capture lower extremities (Fig. 12.4).

Having a plan to streamline the physical examination is important in telehealth examinations due to the limited mobility of the tele-provider's point of view. Just as movies are filmed out of sequence to capture all the needed shots within a camera setup before moving to the next shot setup, a telehealth examination should be viewed with the same "production mindset." Moving and resetting the camera is time-consuming and takes away

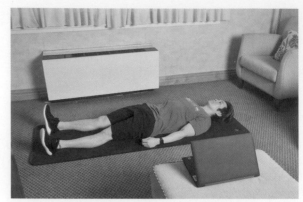
Fig. 12.1 Tilt laptop down if propped up.

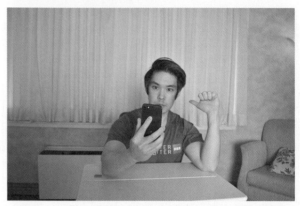
Fig. 12.2 Hold phone for close-up.

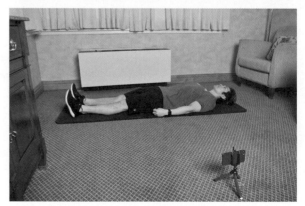
Fig. 12.3 Flip phone horizontally to capture entire body.

from the time the tele-provider will have to examine the patient. To accomplish this, it is recommended to complete all the necessary testing based on a particular position before moving to the next position or camera setup. For example, perform all standing portions of the exam

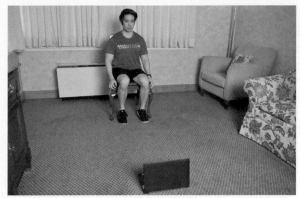

Fig. 12.4 Lower camera position closely to capture lower extremity.

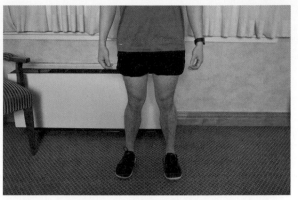

Fig. 12.6 Standing focused view of lower extremties.

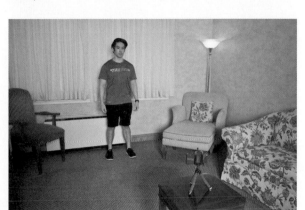

Fig. 12.5 Standing camera setup.

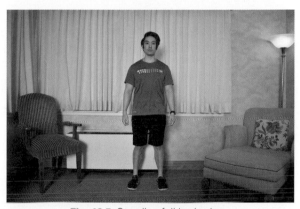

Fig. 12.7 Standing full body view.

first. Have the patient change direction to capture different planes of view. Add a chair and tilt the camera down in its setup to frame the new shot, then turn the chair to capture a lateral view. Lastly, adjust the camera setup to capture any lying positions. Because this is not the usual process for in-person examinations, it takes practice to master this art.

Standing

Bring the camera farther away to better capture the entire body. You can tilt the camera to isolate body regions. Have the patient change directions within the setup to capture different angles and planes of movement (Figs. 12.5, 12.6, 12.7).

Sitting

Angle the camera and place it at the same level as the desired body region to enhance views (Figs. 12.8, 12.9, 12.10, 12.11).

Supine

Elevate the camera to improve the vantage point for comparing left- and right-sided movements (Figs. 12.12, 12.13).

A lower camera may provide better views of unilateral movements (Figs. 12.14, 12.15).

Side Lying

Elevate the camera to improve the vantage point for deviations outside the frontal plane (Figs. 12.16, 12.17).

A lower camera may provide better views of extremity motion (Figs. 12.18, 12.19).

Prone

Position the camera horizontally to improve the view of the full body (Figs. 12.20, 12.21).

All supine, side-lying, and prone exercises may be conducted on a bed, but consider surface stability (Figs. 12.22, 12.23).

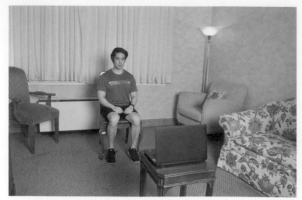

Fig. 12.8 Sitting camera setup for full body view.

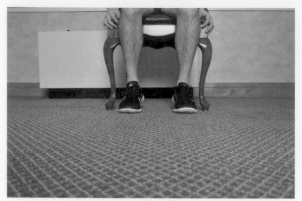

Fig. 12.11 Sitting focused view of lower extremities.

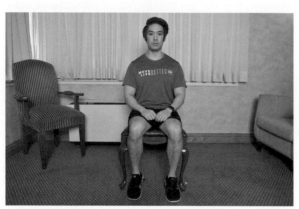

Fig. 12.9 Sitting full body view.

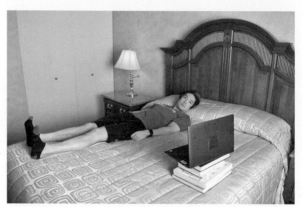

Fig. 12.12 Supine camera setup for full body view.

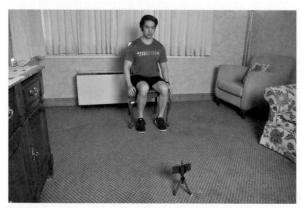

Fig. 12.10 Sitting camera setup for focused view of lower extremities.

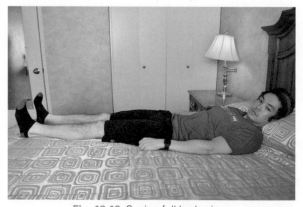

Fig. 12.13 Supine full body view.

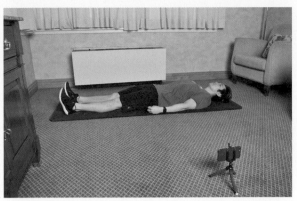

Fig. 12.14 Supine camera setup for unilateral movements.

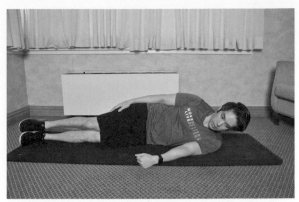

Fig. 12.17 Side-lying elevated view for movements outside frontal plane.

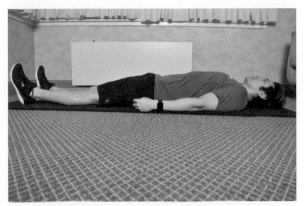

Fig. 12.15 Supine unilateral movement view.

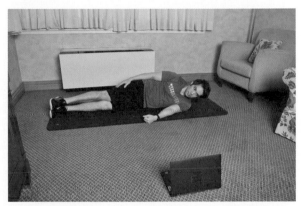

Fig. 12.18 Side-lying floor camera setup for focused movement.

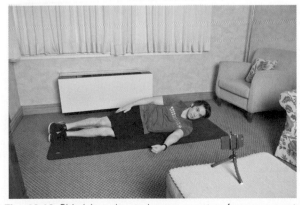

Fig. 12.16 Side-lying elevated camera setup for movements outside frontal plane.

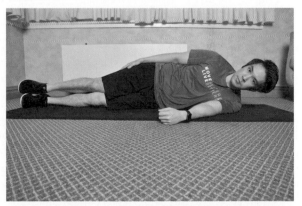

Fig. 12.19 Side-lying floor view for focused movement.

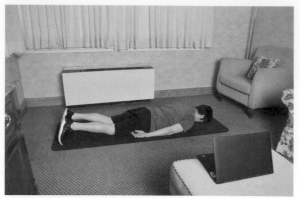

Fig. 12.20 Prone camera setup for full body view.

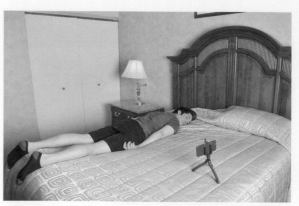

Fig. 12.22 Prone camera setup for full body view in bed.

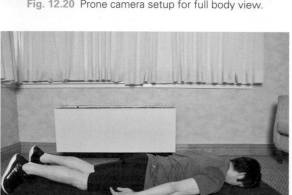

Fig. 12.21 Prone full body view.

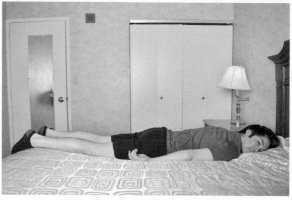

Fig. 12.23 Prone full body view in bed.

TELEHEALTH PHYSICAL EXAM

Telehealth Safety Considerations

Given the limitations of telehealth, a comprehensive sub-jective examination is of the utmost importance to deter-mine whether the patient is appropriate for telehealth assessment. The AAMC has developed competencies regarding patient safety and appropriate use of telehealth, which are presented in the box below.

The subjective examination starts with a thorough red flag evaluation to best triage this patient. Thus, prior to the examina-tion, it is vital to determine whether the patient is appropriate for telehealth assessment. Should there be red flags, they should be evaluated urgently in person with appropriate imaging.

There also may be risk factors and specific circum-stances of the patient or patient population being exam-ined that may not be red flags but indicate that telehealth is not optimal or safe for that patient. Using a tool, or specific

AAMC Telehealth Competencies Domain 1: Patient Safety and Appropriate Use of Telehealth		
Entering residency (recent medical school graduate)	**Entering practice (recent residency graduate)**	**Experienced faculty physician (3–5 years post-residency)**
1a. Explains to patients and caregivers the uses, limita-tions, and benefits of tele-health—that is, the use of electronic communications technology to provide care at a distance	1b. Explains and adapts practice in the context of the limitations and benefits of telehealth	1c. Role models and teaches how to practice telehealth, mitigate risks of providing care at a distance, and assess methods for improvement

AAMC Telehealth Competencies Domain 1: Patient Safety and Appropriate Use of Telehealth—cont'd

Entering residency (recent medical school graduate)	Entering practice (recent residency graduate)	Experienced faculty physician (3–5 years post-residency)
2a. Works with diverse patients and caregivers to determine patient and caregiver access to technology to incorporate telehealth into patient care during real or simulated encounters	2b. Works with diverse patients and caregivers to evaluate and remedy patient and practice barriers to incorporating telehealth into patient care (e.g., access to and comfort with technology)	2c. Role models and teaches how to partner with diverse patients and caregivers in the use of telehealth
3a. Explains to patients and caregivers the roles and responsibilities of team members in telehealth encounters regardless of modality	3b. Demonstrates understanding of all roles and works as a team member when practicing telehealth regardless of modality	3c. Coordinates, implements, and evaluates the effectiveness of the telehealth team regardless of modality
4a. Describes when patient safety is at risk, including when and how to escalate care during a telehealth encounter (e.g., converts to in-person visit or emergency response)	4b. Prepares for and escalates care when patient safety is at risk during a telehealth encounter (e.g., converts to in-person visit or emergency response)	4c. Role models and teaches how to assess patient safety during a telehealth encounter, including preparing for and escalating care when patient safety is at risk

AAMC. (2021). *Telehealth competencies across the learning continuum.* AAMC New and Emerging Areas in Medicine Series. Washington, DC: AAMC.

TABLE 12.4   Musculoskeletal Exam: Body Regions

Spine: cervical and thoracic spine
Spine: lumbar
Shoulder
Elbow, wrist, and hand
Hip
Knee
Ankle and foot

inclusion or exclusion criteria, is a strategy to ensure only appropriate patients are included.

When performing a telehealth visit, it is of utmost importance to confirm the address where the patient is located. Should there be an emergency in which the patient falls or becomes unresponsive, alerting emergency services to the patient's location will be vital. While performing telehealth exams, it is not advised to overly challenge patients with a fall risk with balance testing or any technique that would be guarded by a clinician in the clinic.

As with tools for inclusion into telehealth participation, should a patient's condition change there should be criteria that indicate when a patient should stop telehealth and be referred for in-person care. This may be for safety reasons or when telehealth care is not sufficient to meet the care needs of that patient at that time.

Exam Regions

A musculoskeletal physical examination through telehealth can be subdivided into body regions, with a focus on a specific region based on the indication for the exam (Table 12.4).

Core Exam

The structure of the core exam for all body regions should include visual examination, functional movement assessment, pain identification, ROM, neuromotor assessment, and special tests. Common portions of each core exam are detailed below. The core exam is followed by specific body region red flag considerations that are needed to provide telehealth care safely. Advanced diagnostic considerations are provided to assist in further evaluating the patient.

Visual Examination

The tele-provider should inspect the region for presence of a scar, an incision, ecchymosis, rash, erythema, atrophy, abnormal posture, edema, or deformity. Instructions may be to:
- "Please stand facing the camera so I can see the front of your elbow."
- "Now, turn sideways so I can see the outside of your injured elbow."

TABLE 12.5   **General Range-of-Motion Assessments Using Functional Movements Which Provide an Assumption of Approximate Range of Motion**

Motion	Position	Assessment	Assumption
Hip flexion	Sit to stand	Arising from a chair (16″ chair)	112°
Hip external rotation	Seated	Ankle on contralateral knee putting on shoe	61° (±12°)
Hip adduction	Seated	Knee on contralateral knee putting on shoe	8° (±10°)
Knee flexion	Seated	Ankle on contralateral knee putting on shoe	103° (±6°)

- "Stand facing the camera so I can see you from your knees up and examine your posture."
- "Now do a quarter turn to the right so I can see you from the side."

Functional Movement Assessment

The tele-provider should ask the patient to walk toward and away from the camera and then from side to side. This allows the tele-provider to assess for gait dysfunctions such as antalgic (pain with weight bearing which results in a limp) or steppage gait (increased hip flexion to clear foot during swing phase of gait; this is common with foot drop). Instructions may be to:
- "Stand with your feet shoulder-width apart so I can see your trunk, hip, and knee alignment."
- "Walk directly toward the camera to your starting position and repeat this several times."

Pain Identification

The tele-provider should ask whether pain is present and if so, the specific location and type. Ask the patient to point to the painful area with instructions such as "Where specifically is your pain? Please point to the location using one finger." Ask about feelings of numbness, burning, or tingling. In addition, consider asking whether activities (sitting, running, walking, etc.) worsen or improve symptoms.

Range of Motion

The tele-provider should ask patients to perform bending, flexing, and rotational motions of the involved body region. For general ROM assessment, use functional movements that provide an assumption of approximate ROM (Table 12.5). Instructions may be to:
- "Move approximately 10 feet away from the camera. Turn to the side with your involved shoulder closer to the camera. Bring both arms up as high as you can." (Fig. 12.24)
- "Face the camera. Bring both of your arms out to the side as high as they can go." (Fig. 12.25)

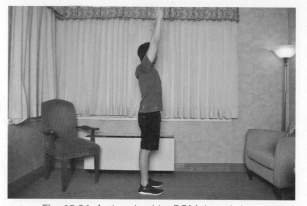

Fig. 12.24 Active shoulder ROM: lateral view.

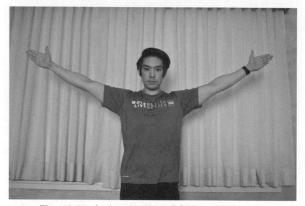

Fig. 12.25 Active shoulder ROM: anterior view.

Neuromotor Assessment

The tele-provider should ask whether the patient is feeling any weakness with any particular movements. If there is weakness, additional testing may be required to better identify the specific dysfunction. With **manual muscle testing** (MMT) specific strength testing, if full ROM is present

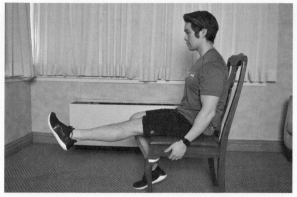

Fig. 12.26 "While sitting, kick your leg out in front of you. Return to the starting position then march your knee up as high as it can go."

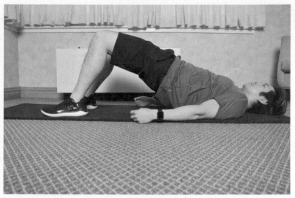

Fig. 12.28 "Bend both knees up so your feet are on the ground. Lift your buttocks in the air and hold for the requested amount of time, then return to the start position."

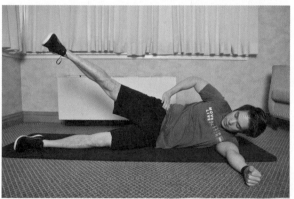

Fig. 12.27 "Lie on your uninvolved side, facing the camera. Keep your involved leg straight and lift it in the air."

against gravity, MMT grade is at least 3/5 (Hislop et al., 2013). Patient can perform self over-pressure to grade greater than 3/5. Fig. 12.26 shows knee extension to assess for quadriceps strength against gravity, and Fig. 12.27 shows hip abduction strength against gravity. Functional strength assessments can suffice in lieu of traditional MMT. Fig. 12.28 shows hip extension strength from a bridge motion.

Special Tests

These are specific advanced diagnostic tests, per body region or nature of complaint, to assist in confirming a diagnosis or with differential diagnosis (Magee, 2014).

Body Region-Specific Red Flags and Special Tests
Hip

Examples of red flags for the hip exam are shown in Table 12.6. It is important to rule out lumbar spine pathology for lower extremity exams, as symptoms in the lower extremity may originate from the lumbar spine (Magee, 2014). To

TABLE 12.6 Hip Assessment Red Flags	
Red flag questions	**Suspected diagnosis**
Have you sustained recent trauma resulting in pain or disability?	Undetermined
Are you experiencing difficulty or change with your bowel/bladder habits? Any numbness in your groin region?	Cauda equina, urological pathology
Are you experiencing unrelenting pain that does not change? Unplanned weight loss or history of cancer?	Cancer
Have you recently noticed a pronounced pulse in your stomach?	Abdominal aortic aneurism
Any recent increase in your activity levels, exercise, or training volumes related to your pain?	Stress fracture
Any recent illness, fever, or chills associated with your hip pain?	Infection

Source: HSS MD tele guide.

perform lumbar screen, have the patient flex, extend, rotate, and laterally bend their lumbar spine to see if symptoms are reproduced. For advanced diagnostic considerations, common hip special tests which may be modified for telehealth

TABLE 12.7 Knee Assessment Red Flags

Red flag questions	Suspected diagnosis
Have you recently experienced trauma?	Fracture, dislocation
Did your symptoms start after an increase in exercise?	Stress reaction
Do you have calf pain with redness and/or swelling?	Deep vein thrombosis
Have you experienced a recent fever or chills?	Infection

TABLE 12.8 Ankle and Foot Assessment Red Flags

Question	Suspected diagnosis
Have you recently experienced trauma?	Fracture, tendon rupture
Did your symptoms start after an increase in exercise?	Stress fracture
Do you have calf pain with redness and/or swelling?	Deep vein thrombosis
Have you noticed any discoloration or feelings of coldness?	Vascular compromise
Have you experienced recent fever or chills?	Infection

TABLE 12.9 Lumbar Spine Assessment Red Flags

Red flag questions	Suspected diagnosis
Have you sustained recent trauma resulting in pain or disability?	Undetermined
Are you experiencing abdominal pain? Pain related to meals?	Gallbladder, stomach
Are you experiencing difficulty with bowel/bladder? Any numbness in your groin region?	Cauda equina
Are you experiencing unrelenting pain that does not change? Unplanned weight loss or history of cancer?	Cancer
Have you recently noticed a pronounced pulse in your stomach?	Abdominal aortic aneurism
Any recent illness, fever, or chills associated with your back pain?	Infection

include the Flexion, Adduction, Internal Rotation (FADIR) (Philippon et al., 2007) and flexion abduction external rotation (FABER) tests for femoro-acetabular impingement (Shanmugaraj et al., 2020), and the Thomas test for hip flexor tightness (Peeler & Anderson, 2008).

Knee

Examples of red flags for the knee exam are shown in Table 12.7. For advanced diagnostic considerations, common knee special tests which may be modified for telehealth include the flexion McMurray test for meniscus tear (Greis et al., 2002), step down test (Lopes Ferreira et al., 2019) or single leg squat (Herrington, 2014) for patellofemoral pathology.

Ankle and Foot

Examples of red flags for the ankle and foot exam are shown in Table 12.8. For advanced diagnostic considerations,

common foot and ankle special tests which may be modified for telehealth include the Thompson test for Achilles rupture (Mazzone & McCue, 2002) (caregiver required), single-leg balance test for ankle sprain (Trojian & McKeag, 2006), Homan's sign for deep vein thrombosis (Levi et al., 1999), and the Windlass test for plantar fasciitis (Bolgla & Malone, 2004).

Lumbar Spine

Examples of red flags for the lumbar exam are shown in Table 12.9. For advanced diagnostic considerations, common special tests which may be modified for telehealth are the slump and straight leg raise (SLR) tests for lumbar radiculopathy or stenosis (Majlesi et al., 2008).

Shoulder

Examples of red flags for the shoulder exam are shown in Table 12.10. It is important to rule out cervical spine pathology for upper extremity exams, as symptoms in the upper extremity may originate from the cervical spine (Magee, 2014). To perform a cervical screen, have the patient flex, extend, rotate, and laterally bend the cervical spine to see if symptoms are reproduced. For advanced diagnostic considerations,

TABLE 12.10   Shoulder Assessment Red Flags

Question	Suspected diagnosis
Have you recently experienced trauma?	Fracture, dislocation
Do you notice constant painful arm swelling, redness, or warmth?	Deep vein thrombosis
Are your symptoms unchanged with movements?	Cancer
Are your symptoms provoked by exertion despite not moving your arm?	Cardiac
Are your symptoms provoked by neck movements?	Cervical radiculopathy

TABLE 12.11   Elbow, Wrist, and Hand Assessment Red Flags

Question	Suspected diagnosis
Have you sustained recent trauma resulting in pain or disability?	Undetermined
Do you notice constant painful arm swelling, redness, or warmth?	Deep vein thrombosis
Are your symptoms unchanged with movements?	Cancer
Are your symptoms provoked by exertion despite not moving your arm?	Cardiac
Are your symptoms provoked by neck movements?	Cervical radiculopathy

common shoulder special tests which may be modified for telehealth include the Hawkins/Kennedy test for rotator cuff impingement (Hawkins & Kennedy, 1980), drop arm test for rotator cuff tear (Mitchell et al., 2005), cross body test for acromioclavicular joint dysfunction (van Riet & Bell, 2011), apprehension test for shoulder instability (Farber et al., 2006), speeds test for biceps tendinopathy (Kim et al., 2020), and Roos test for thoracic outlet syndrome (Hixson et al., 2017).

Elbow, Wrist, and Hand

Examples of red flags for the elbow, wrist, and hand exam are shown in Table 12.11. Perform a cervical screen to rule out cervical spine pathology. For advanced diagnostic considerations, common special tests which may be modified for telehealth for the elbow are Maudsley's test for lateral epicondylitis (Duncan et al., 2019); for the wrist is Finkelstein's test for de Quervain's tenosynovitis (Dawson & Mudgal, 2010); for the hand is Phalen's sign for carpal tunnel syndrome (Kuschner et al., 1992).

Cervical and Thoracic Spine

Examples of red flags for the cervical and thoracic spine exam are shown in Table 12.12. For advanced diagnostic considerations, common special tests which may be modified for telehealth are Spurling's test (Thoomes et al., 2018) and the upper limb tension test (ULTT) (Ghasemi et al., 2013) for cervical radiculopathy or stenosis.

TABLE 12.12   Cervical and Thoracic Spine Assessment Red Flags

Question	Suspected diagnosis
Have you recently experienced trauma?	Fracture
Have you been experiencing dizziness, nausea, headaches or fainting/drop attacks recently?	CNS lesion, coronary artery disease, cervical ligament damage
Have you experienced recent changes in vision, hearing, or swallowing?	CNS lesion
Have you had recent difficulty with walking or falling?	Myelopathy, CNS lesion
Have you experienced a recent fever or chills?	Infection

Postoperative Considerations

For postoperative patients, there are considerations which should be accounted for during a telehealth exam. These considerations include but are not limited to: incision or dressing status, presence of precautions, restricted movements, ROM limits, signs of deep vein thrombus or pulmonary embolism, weight-bearing allowance.

For patients who are immediately postoperative, the core examination should be modified to include an observational, neurovascular, and screening assessment of the associated body region. For subacute and chronic phases, ROM and strength testing will be dependent on the procedure performed and the postoperative timeframe. The purpose of this examination is to identify any concerns that would require additional in-person follow-up and evaluation.

TELEHEALTH USE CASES

Telehealth has been emerging slowly over time as a medium for providing patient care. In March 2020 the COVID-19 pandemic highlighted the value of telehealth to facilitate social distancing and quarantine. At Hospital for Special Surgery in New York City, there were two small telehealth programs prior to the pandemic, which performed fewer than 1500 patient visits in 2019. Due to COVID-19, the hospital swiftly expanded its telehealth care programs and infrastructure to allow for necessary patient care, which resulted in the hospital performing over 100,000 telehealth visits from March 2020 through November 2020. This allowed the interdisciplinary team of physicians, nurses, therapists, physician assistants, nurse practitioners, social workers, and others to care for all types of patients, whether they were new or existing, surgical or nonsurgical. The hospital's telehealth care is provided through its secure electronic health record which allows all disciplines to document in a central location, facilitating enhanced interdisciplinary communication and teamwork.

An example of a telehealth interdisciplinary team is the hospital's postacute programs. Following a patient's discharge from the hospital, the physical therapist (PT) treats the patient through telehealth. Any questions or issues the patient has that are out of the scope of a PT are directed by the PT to the medical team of physicians, nurses, and physician assistants, who contact that patient via phone, a virtual visit, or an in-person visit to address the issue. Any social-related issues are communicated to the social work team. All communication and intervention is documented in the patient's electronic record so that other providers engaging in care with the patient have access to the patient's history.

Relevant Guidelines

Telehealth Physical Therapy Assessment: HSS Rehabilitation Telehealth Evaluation Guidelines for Musculoskeletal Physical Therapy
- Full orthopedic assessment: Magee (2014)
- Full orthopedic assessment: Miller's Review of Orthopaedics, eighth Edition.

SUMMARY

- Musculoskeletal telehealth care requires factoring in many considerations that are not present with in-person care, to ensure quality and effectiveness.
- Tele-providers should be prepared with the necessary training, understanding of general telehealth considerations, and ability to perform a telehealth physical exam while understanding telehealth safety considerations.
- Patients should be educated to be prepared for the visits in advance to minimize disturbances and maximize time with the tele-provider.
- Camera setup and considerations are vital for a successful exam, as this is the only way for the tele-provider to visualize the patient.

KEY POINTS

- The process of a telehealth musculoskeletal assessment is not synonymous with conducting an in-person assessment.
- Proper lighting and camera setup are needed for the tele-provider to effectively visualize and assess the patient.
- Tele-providers and patients should prepare the environment in advance to maximize clinical time and minimize delays.
- Not all patients should receive telehealth care. Providers should understand safety considerations, red flags, and when to refer for in-person assessment.
- The core exam comprises visual examination, functional movement assessment, pain identification, range of motion, neuromotor assessment, and special tests.
- Postsurgical considerations are important to ensure proper care and identify any concerns that would require additional in-person follow-up and evaluation.

REFERENCES

AAMC. (2021). *Telehealth competencies across the learning continuum. AAMC New and Emerging Areas in Medicine Series.* Washington, DC: AAMC.

Bolgla, L. A., & Malone, T. R. (2004). Plantar fasciitis and the windlass mechanism: A biomechanical link to clinical practice. *Journal of Athletic Training, 39*(1), 77–82.

Dawson, C., & Mudgal, C. S. (2010). Staged description of the Finkelstein test. *Journal of Hand Surgery (American Volume), 35*(9), 1513–1515. https://doi.org/10.1016/j.jhsa.2010.05.022.

Duncan, J., Duncan, R., Bansal, S., et al. (2019). Lateral epicondylitis: The condition and current management strategies. *British Journal of Hospital Medicine, 80*(11), 647–651. https://doi.org/10.12968/hmed.2019.80.11.647.

Farber, A. J., Castillo, R., Clough, M., et al. (2006). Clinical assessment of three common tests for traumatic anterior shoulder instability. *The Journal of Bone and Joint Surgery, 88*(7), 1467–1474. https://doi.org/10.2106/JBJS.E.00594.

Ghasemi, M., Golabchi, K., Mousavi, S. A., et al. (2013). The value of provocative tests in diagnosis of cervical radiculopathy. *Journal of Research in Medical Sciences, 18*(Suppl. 1), S35–S38.

Greis, P. E., Bardana, D. D., Holmstrom, M. C., et al. (2002). Meniscal injury: I. Basic science and evaluation. *Journal of the American Academy of Orthopaedic Surgeons, 10*(3), 168–176. https://doi.org/10.5435/00124635-200205000-00003.

Hawkins, R. J., & Kennedy, J. C. (1980). Impingement syndrome in athletes. *The American Journal of Sports Medicine, 8*(3), 151–158. https://doi.org/10.1177/036354658000800302.

Herrington, L. (2014). Knee valgus angle during single leg squat and landing in patellofemoral pain patients and controls. *The Knee, 21*(2), 514–517. https://doi.org/10.1016/j.knee.2013.11.011.

Hislop, H., Avers, D., & Brown, M. (2013). *Daniels and Worthingham's muscle testing: Techniques of manual examination and performance testing* (9th ed.). St. Louis, MO: Elsevier Saunders.

Hixson, K. M., Horris, H. B., McLeod, T. C. V., et al. (2017). The diagnostic accuracy of clinical diagnostic tests for thoracic outlet syndrome. *Journal of Sport Rehabilitation, 26*(5), 459–465. https://doi.org/10.1123/jsr.2016-0051.

HSS Rehabilitation. (2020). *Telehealth evaluation guidelines for musculoskeletal physical therapy. Independently published.* Amazon.

Kim, J., Nam, J. H., Kim, Y., et al. (2020). Long head of the biceps tendon tenotomy versus subpectoral tenodesis in rotator cuff repair. *Clinics in Orthopedic Surgery, 12*(3), 371–378. https://doi.org/10.4055/cios19168.

Kuschner, S. H., Ebramzadeh, E., Johnson, D., et al. (1992). Tinel's sign and Phalen's test in carpal tunnel syndrome. *Orthopedics, 15*(11), 1297–1302.

Levi, M., Hart, W., & Büller, H. R. (1999). [Physical examination--the significance of Homan's sign]. *Nederlands Tijdschrift Voor Geneeskunde, 143*(37), 1861–1863.

Lopes Ferreira, C., Barton, G., Delgado Borges, L., et al. (2019). Step down tests are the tasks that most differentiate the kinematics of women with patellofemoral pain compared to asymptomatic controls. *Gait & Posture, 72*, 129–134. https://doi.org/10.1016/j.gaitpost.2019.05.023.

Magee, D. J. (2014). *Orthopedic physical assessment* (6th ed.). St. Louis, MO: Elsevier. Saunders.

Majlesi, J., Togay, H., Unalan, H., et al. (2008). The sensitivity and specificity of the slump and the straight leg raising tests in patients with lumbar disc herniation. *Journal of Clinical Rheumatology, 14*(2), 87–91. https://doi.org/10.1097/RHU.0b013e31816b2f99.

Mazzone, M. F., & McCue, T. (2002). Common conditions of the Achilles tendon. *American Family Physician, 65*(9), 1805–1810.

Mitchell, C., Adebajo, A., Hay, E., et al. (2005). Shoulder pain: Diagnosis and management in primary care. *BMJ, 331*(7525), 1124–1128. https://doi.org/10.1136/bmj.331.7525.1124.

Peeler, J. D., & Anderson, J. E. (2008). Reliability limits of the modified Thomas test for assessing rectus femoris muscle flexibility about the knee joint. *Journal of Athletic Training, 43*(5), 470–476. https://doi.org/10.4085/1062-6050-43.5.470.

Philippon, M. J., Maxwell, R. B., Johnston, T. L., et al. (2007). Clinical presentation of femoroacetabular impingement. *Knee Surgery Sports Traumatology Arthroscopy, 15*(8), 1041–1047. https://doi.org/10.1007/s00167-007-0348-2.

Shanmugaraj, A., Shell, J. R., Horner, N. S., et al. (2020). How useful is the flexion-adduction-internal rotation test for diagnosing femoroacetabular impingement: A systematic review. *Clinical Journal of Sport Medicine, 30*(1), 76–82. https://doi.org/10.1097/JSM.0000000000000575.

Theraband. *Theraband professional non-latex resistance bands.* https://www.theraband.com/theraband-professional-non-latex-resistance-bands-25-yard-roll.html. [Accessed 1 November 2021].

Thoomes, E. J., van Geest, S., van der Windt, D. A., et al. (2018). Value of physical tests in diagnosing cervical radiculopathy: A systematic review. *The Spine Journal, 18*(1), 179–189. https://doi.org/10.1016/j.spinee.2017.08.241.

Trojian, T. H., & McKeag, D. B. (2006). Single leg balance test to identify risk of ankle sprains. *British Journal of Sports Medicine, 40*(7), 610–613;discussion 613. https://doi.org/10.1136/bjsm.2005.024356.

van Riet, R. P., & Bell, S. N. (2011). Clinical evaluation of acromioclavicular joint pathology: Sensitivity of a new test. *Journal of Shoulder and Elbow Surgery, 20*(1), 73–76. https://doi.org/10.1016/j.jse.2010.05.023.

INDEX

Note: Page numbers followed by "f" indicate figures, "t" indicate tables and "b" indicate boxes.